Polyvagal Theory

Becoming Ph Balanced in an Unbalanced World

(A Practical Guide to Starting Developing and Sustaining a Therapy Practice)

Edwin Mays

I0089851

Published By **Phil Dawson**

Edwin Mays

All Rights Reserved

Polyvagal Theory: Becoming Ph Balanced in an Unbalanced World (A Practical Guide to Starting Developing and Sustaining a Therapy Practice)

ISBN   978-1-7776028-8-8

Published By **Phil Dawson**

ISBN   978-1-7776028-8-8

No part of this guidebook shall be reproduced in any form without permission in writing from the publisher except in the case of brief quotations embodied in critical articles or reviews.

Legal & Disclaimer

Table Of Contents

Chapter 1: Discovering The Polyvagal Theory

As we transition into the coronary heart of our exploration, it is vital to recount the genesis of the Polyvagal Theory, its important architect, Stephen Porges, and the indelible mark it has left at the landscape of psychotherapy and beyond. The Polyvagal Theory emerged no longer simply as a theoretical framework but as a lens via which we should higher apprehend the nuanced interaction among our physiological structures and our emotional evaluations.

The narrative of the Polyvagal Theory started out out to unfold within the past due 20th century at the same time as Stephen Porges, a pioneering mind in the realm of psychophysiology, set forth on a quest to demystify the complex interactions among the autonomic anxious tool (ANS) and our emotional and social behaviors. The concept, grounded in meticulous studies and eager assertion, unveiled a unique attitude on how our worried device operates, in particular emphasizing the position of the vagus nerve.

Porges' investigations led to the revealing of the "polyvagal mindset," a time period now synonymous with a more holistic and included expertise of human feelings, stress responses, and interpersonal interactions. This mind-set shed moderate on the mechanisms underlying our reactions to pressure, our capacity for social engagement, and the pathways thru which we are able to cultivate a sense of protection and balance in our lives.

DISCOVERING THE POLYVAGAL THEORY

In the place of psychotherapy and neurobiology, theories and frameworks shape the bedrock of understanding complicated human behaviors, emotions, and interpersonal interactions. One such groundbreaking framework is the Polyvagal Theory, introduced with the aid of manner of Dr. Stephen Porges within the late 20th century. This concept has not most effective broadened the horizons of expertise regarding the autonomic anxious tool but additionally bridged the as soon as reputedly faraway fields of neurobiology and psychotherapy.

DEFINING THE POLYVAGAL THEORY

The Polyvagal Theory elucidates a completely particular interplay among our hectic system and our emotional or social demeanor. At its middle, it unveils the functioning of the vagus nerve, a cranial nerve that interfaces with our coronary coronary heart, lungs, and digestive tract, orchestrating a myriad of important functions pivotal for our survival and nicely-being.

Dr. Stephen Porges, through meticulous research, determined that the vagus nerve isn't surely a solitary, uniform entity but a complicated, branching community capable of a myriad of capabilities. His exploration brought about the identity of a "ventral vagal complicated" this is related to our social engagement behaviors and a "dorsal vagal complicated" this is often brought on beneath excessive pressure.

In easy terms, the Polyvagal Theory permits decipher the physiological underpinnings of our reactions, whether or not or no longer it's far a peaceful, composed response in a socially attractive scenario, or a fight-or-flight response underneath threat. It extends past simply explaining the ones reactions, losing light on how our body shape is deeply intertwined with our emotional states, and in the end, our highbrow health.

The idea ushers in an technology of information that our our our bodies aren't sincerely vessels, however dynamic, responsive entities continuously interacting with their environment. It posits that our capability for social interactions, our ability to attune to others, and our propensity towards both a stable, social engagement or a protecting stance is largely modulated through the workings of the vagus nerve.

Furthermore, the principle elucidates the concept of "neuroception," a term coined with the aid of the use of Porges to provide an explanation for how our nervous system discerns cues of protection, threat, or lifestyles chance from our surroundings, even out of doors of aware interest. This subconscious mechanism substantially affects our interactions, our perception of protection, and our potential to hook up with others.

The Polyvagal Theory could no longer in reality prevent at explaining those physiological mechanisms; it opens doorways to a plethora of restoration interventions. By understanding the deep-seated physiological roots of many highbrow fitness problems, therapists, and those alike, can better navigate the roads to recuperation and private growth. Moreover, it lays a sturdy foundation for integrating neurophysiological insights with psychotherapeutic practices, that is important for evolving more powerful healing interventions.

The insights from the Polyvagal Theory have reverberated via the corridors of psychotherapy, providing a clean lens to apprehend and cope with the difficult interplay between the mind and the frame. It extends an invitation to discover a deeper knowledge of ourselves, fostering a adventure of self-discovery and restoration.

THE SCIENTIFIC BASIS OF POLYVAGAL THEORY

The Polyvagal Theory, conceived with the useful resource of Dr. Stephen Porges, is a pioneering narrative that entwines the cloth of physiological skills with the tapestry of mental studies. At its middle, it endeavors to clarify the mechanisms through which our stressful tool interfaces with our emotions and behaviors, mainly inside the realm of social engagement and reactions to threats or protection.

The concept is grounded within the exploration of the vagus nerve and its myriad competencies. This nerve is corresponding to a bi-directional conversation superhighway between the thoughts and the frame. Its tentacles attain out to numerous organs, orchestrating a symphony of responses that echo via the canyons of our inner physiological landscape, resonating inside the out of doors theater of our social interactions.

Polyvagal Theory takes its call from the vagus nerve which, as illustrated inside the previous subchapter, has a twin, or as an opportunity 'poly'-vagal, shape. The ventral and dorsal branches of the vagus nerve shape the crux of this concept, every with its high-quality role in the dance of survival and social engagement.

The technology within the back of this principle is rich and multi-dimensional, encompassing the geographical areas of neurophysiology, psychology, and behavioral era. It delves into the nuances of the manner our nervous device, thru the vagus nerve, impacts our functionality to apprehend and respond to the sector spherical us.

At a microscopic diploma, the workings of the vagus nerve are not something short of awe-inspiring. Its functionality to modulate heart charge, manipulate breath, and have an effect on digestion is a testimony to the inherent know-how housed inner our physiological structure. The ventral vagal pathway, associated with the 'social engagement system', opens the doorways to connection, communique, and feelings of protection. Conversely, the dorsal vagal pathway comes into play on the same time because the device perceives risk, orchestrating a retreat into conservation and self-protection.

The Polyvagal Theory additionally introduces a ultra-modern lexicon into the communicate amongst frame and thoughts. Terms like 'neuroception', which refers to how our nervous device scans the surroundings for cues of protection or chance, and 'co-regulation', it without a doubt is the interaction of worried systems amongst people in a social context, grow to be primary difficulty topics on this narrative.

Furthermore, the principle explores the idea of 'physiological u . S .' and its effect on our behavior, emotions, and ability to connect to others. It proposes that our physiological state, modulated through the use of the vagus nerve, units the diploma for the way we revel in and have interaction with the area.

The Polyvagal Theory is not simply a scientific idea, but a lens thru which we are able to view and make feel of human revel in. It gives a framework for knowledge the physiological underpinnings of highbrow health troubles, trauma, and recuperation. It's a bridge that connects the frequently segregated islands of body and mind, supplying a holistic, integrative mind-set that holds promise for a deeper knowledge of the human circumstance.

In unfolding the scientific tapestry of the Polyvagal Theory, we inch in the direction of a holistic comprehension of methods our internal herbal narrative impacts our outer social narrative. It's a assignment into the center of human experience, an exploration that ensures to shed light on the mysteries of our existence and offer a stable basis for the unfolding discourse inside the chapters to examine.

Through the lens of Polyvagal Theory, we start to see the difficult choreography of frame and mind in a present day slight, a revelation that beckons a deeper exploration into the harmonies and discords that compose the symphony of human revel in.

THE VAGUS NERVE: YOUR BODY'S COMPASS

At the coronary coronary coronary heart of the Polyvagal Theory lies the vagus nerve, a wonder of nature that acts as a compass within our our our bodies, guiding our responses to the area round us. The vagus nerve isn't always only a bodily shape, however a portal into the complicated dance of body and thoughts, emotions and cognition.

A silent manual, the vagus nerve is your frame's compass amidst the seas of life's stories. It's a communication highway, linking the narrative of your body to the narrative of your experience. It is thru this important nerve that we start to remedy the tapestry of the Polyvagal Theory.

THE VAGUS NERVE extends its tendrils from the brainstem right all the way down to the stomach, touching the coronary coronary heart and lungs along its descent, like a moderate whisper flowing thru the middle of our being. It's the longest cranial nerve, and its name, because of this 'wandering' in Latin, aptly describes its enormous achieve all through numerous organs.

The branches of the vagus nerve, the ventral and dorsal, are the key players in this narrative. The ventral vagal complicated is frequently seen due to the fact the protagonist, promoting social engagement and fostering feelings of safety and connection. On the alternative component, the dorsal vagal complicated may be taken into consideration because the vigilant father or mother, ready to spring into motion in the course of instances of perceived chance, mobilizing the body's defensive techniques.

However, it's miles an oversimplification to sturdy those branches in handiest black and white sunglasses. The interaction between them is a nuanced communicate, an ongoing conversation that shapes our belief of protection, threat, and life's myriad conditions. They are the duo venture the orchestra of our autonomic responses, playing the symphony of our every day evaluations.

The ventral vagal pathway allows the harmonies of our social interactions, allowing us to study and respond to cues from our surroundings and from others. It's a bearer of peace, supporting to calm the internal storms, bearing in thoughts a rhythm of ease and go together with the drift in our interactions. On the alternative hand, the dorsal vagal pathway orchestrates the more primal rhythms of survival, marshaling sources in times of need, but it too has its location in the symphony of our being.

The vagus nerve's capability to figure amongst a tune of protection and a tune of chance is pivotal. This discernment, termed 'neuroception' via Dr. Porges, is an subconscious method, however it shapes our aware memories in profound methods. It's the melody that underpins our emotions of safety or chance, of connection or isolation.

Delving deeper into the essence of the vagus nerve is comparable to tuning into the diffused but profound rhythms of our body, which in flip, echo the rhythms of our lived critiques. It's a voyage into the coronary heart of the Polyvagal Theory, into understanding how this silent guide, this frame's compass, shapes our interactions with the world, our relationships, and ultimately, our know-how of self.

As we venture in addition into the geographical areas of the Polyvagal Theory, the vagus nerve is probably our manual, our compass, leading us thru the landscapes of neurobiology and psychology, dropping light on how our inner frame structure impacts our outer tales.

The narrative of the vagus nerve is a foundational stone in our exploration, illuminating the pathways thru which we recognize and navigate our life. Through comprehending the vagus nerve, we are not sincerely understanding a physiological shape, but unlocking a doorway to a greater profound knowledge of our being in the international, placing the diploma for the upcoming exploration of the Polyvagal Theory inside the next chapters of this narrative.

Chapter 2: Neurodivergence

UNDERSTANDING NEURODIVERGENT EXPERIENCES

The realm of neurodivergence is as diverse and multifaceted as the people it encompasses. Unraveling the myriad reminiscences of neurodivergent people thru the lens of the Polyvagal Theory not excellent propels us in the course of a deeper comprehension however furthermore fosters a platform for brought empathetic engagements and supportive environments. This exploration is akin to embarking on a voyage right into a good sized ocean of man or woman evaluations, each wave revealing particular kinds of neurophysiological responses and emotional interactions.

The Polyvagal Theory, with its consciousness on the autonomic traumatic gadget, gives a framework to understand the nuanced neurophysiological underpinnings that play out within the lives of neurodivergent people. The vagus nerve, being a cornerstone of this concept, bureaucracy a conduit via which we are able to discover the interplay a number of the thoughts, frame, and social environment.

In the domain of neurodivergence, one may moreover discover that the manner in which the fearful device responds to stimuli, each from inner and outside the body, takes a extremely good pathway. The adaptive strategies employed with the resource of neurodivergent human beings often replicate a unique choreography of neural circuits orchestrated via the vagus nerve.

For example, the reviews of people at the autism spectrum can be illuminated thru the prism of the Polyvagal Theory. The sensory processing peculiarities, social engagement challenges, and the look for protection and comfort can be construed as manifestations of the autonomic anxious device's striving for equilibrium.

Similarly, people with hobby-deficit/hyperactivity ailment (ADHD) show off a one-of-a-type rhythmic dance of neural activations and responses. The Polyvagal lens may unveil how their worried structures have interaction with the milieu of stimuli that envelop them, often important to styles which might be misinterpreted or pathologized.

Moreover, the experiences of people with sensory processing illness, anxiety, despair, and exceptional neurodivergent conditions may be delved into with a Polyvagal mindset. This precept can manual us in recognizing the neurophysiological narratives that underlie the behaviors and responses exhibited through neurodivergent human beings.

Furthermore, the Polyvagal Theory aids in transcending the pathologizing narrative that regularly surrounds neurodivergence. By fostering a language of know-how and recognition, it nudges society within the course of developing nurturing areas that honor the neurophysiological range among us.

THIS EXPLORATION IS NOT about labeling or defining people based totally mostly on their neurodivergent conditions. Rather, it is an invitation to honor the diverse tapestry of human testimonies and to increase our records and empathy in the direction of the neurodivergent community.

The narratives of neurodivergent humans, at the same time as regarded via the Polyvagal lens, turn out to be stories of resilience, variant, and the indomitable spirit of navigating existence in a neurotypical worldwide. Through the ones narratives, we are not best gaining knowledge of approximately the myriad methods in which our apprehensive structures have interaction with the arena however moreover approximately the boundless potential for fostering connections, knowledge, and reputation in the numerous world we inhabit.

REAL-LIFE CASES: POLYVAGAL THEORY IN ACTION

The Polyvagal Theory unveils a dynamic interplay of neurophysiological mechanisms which can be on the middle of our evaluations, in particular for the neurodivergent network. To better recognize its effect and application, allow's delve into actual-life situations in which Polyvagal Theory has been a lens thru which people and professionals have navigated the neurodivergent landscape.

Case 1: Autism and Social Engagement

Jonas, a younger boy diagnosed with Autism Spectrum Disorder (ASD), frequently decided social interactions to be overwhelming. Through the lens of Polyvagal Theory, his therapists must discern that his neurophysiological reaction to social stimuli became dominated through way of his frame's primal need for safety. Recognizing the nuances of the vagal pathways helped tailor interventions that slowly constructed a enjoy of safety, allowing Jonas to navigate social settings with growing ease.

Case 2: ADHD and Self-Regulation

Sophia, a younger grownup with Attention-Deficit/Hyperactivity Disorder (ADHD), struggled with impulsivity and staying focused. Through a Polyvagal-knowledgeable technique, she have become guided to boom a extra recognition of her body's signals. By tuning into her physiological state, she must higher understand whilst she changed into turning into dysregulated and lease strategies to regain a experience of stability.

Case 3: Sensory Processing and Trauma

Liam, who had a records of trauma, exhibited heightened sensitivity to sensory stimuli. Professionals the use of a Polyvagal framework helped Liam apprehend the relationship amongst his sensory processing disturbing conditions and past stressful studies. This information have become instrumental in developing coping techniques that more his resilience and stepped forward his extremely good of lifestyles.

Case 4: Anxiety and Body Awareness

Emma, living with anxiety, determined solace in understanding her reviews via the Polyvagal lens. Gaining perception into how her frightened tool responded to perceived threats allowed her to broaden self-compassion. It moreover fostered a pathway inside the course of reading techniques that would assist alter her physiological usa, thereby reducing the depth and frequency of anxiety episodes.

These times elucidate how a Polyvagal attitude may be transformative. It no longer most effective offers a framework for information person variations however additionally opens avenues for interventions which is probably attuned to the neurophysiological narratives of neurodivergent humans. By embracing the eye encapsulated in the Polyvagal Theory, a road unfolds in the course of extra compassionate and effective manual for the neurodivergent network. This isn't always in reality a theoretical exploration but a call towards adopting a lens that honors the neurodivergent experience in all its complexity and functionality for boom and model.

As we flow into ahead, the insights gleaned from the ones real-life situations will function a scaffold, enriching our discussions on the numerous dimensions of Polyvagal profound implications. By dissecting the nuances in every case, we unfold the layers of expertise critical for formulating holistic techniques which is probably uniquely suitable to every individual's neurodivergent narrative.

In the course of Emma's, Jonas's, Sophia's, and Liam's studies, we witness the functionality for a extra nuanced information and alertness of the Polyvagal Theory. Their tales shed moderate at the pivotal characteristic of protection, connection, and physiological law in navigating the tapestry of neurodivergence. Each tale is a sworn announcement to the transformative power of viewing neurodivergence thru a Polyvagal lens, fostering a weather of reputation, facts, and tailored assist.

The tapestry of interactions most of the neural circuits, as depicted inside the Polyvagal Theory, and the outdoor worldwide, turns into vividly illustrated within the ones cases. It's a communicate between the inner physiological nation-states and the out of doors environments that mould the lived reports of neurodivergent humans. The information and alertness of Polyvagal Theory consequently emerge as a bridge in the route of fostering resilience, self-reputation, and progressed interplay with the area.

Moreover, the ones narratives underscore the significance of a multidisciplinary technique. The interplay some of the intellectual, physiological, and social geographical regions necessitates a collaborative strive amongst professionals from various fields. This collaborative ethos, knowledgeable via the use of the Polyvagal Theory, holds the promise of crafting healing processes which may be as numerous and dynamic because the neurodivergent human beings they will be searching out to assist.

As we venture similarly into the depths of the Polyvagal Theory and its software within the realm of neurodivergence, those real-existence times serve as every a manual and a supply of perception. They invite us to explore, to impeach, and to ascertain a realm of opportunities wherein the neurodivergent community isn't always genuinely understood but is supported in a way that resonates with their innate neurophysiological make-up. In subsequent discussions, the richness of these actual-lifestyles packages will be similarly explored, imparting a well-rounded angle at the multifaceted techniques in which the Polyvagal Theory can be operationalized to decorate the lives of neurodivergent individuals and the groups they're part of. Through this lens, we begin to see now not just the annoying situations, but the significant potential looking for to be unveiled as we align our beneficial useful resource systems with the inherent knowledge of the human frame as elucidated thru the Polyvagal Theory.

ADAPTING POLYVAGAL EXERCISES FOR NEURODIVERGENCE

In navigating the channels of Polyvagal Theory and neurodivergence, the capability for model, particularly within the realm of sporting activities tailored to the neurodivergent network, emerges as a hopeful frontier. The marriage of Polyvagal insights with the numerous opinions of neurodivergent humans paves the manner for a extra inclusive, respectful, and effective method.

The essence of Polyvagal physical games lies in promoting a country of safety, from which the autonomic fearful device can foster a revel in of connection and social engagement. However, what constitutes a 'consistent' surroundings or enjoy can extensively range among neurodivergent humans. The textures of sensory processing, social interactions, and emotional responses are frequently fairly extremely good, requiring a thoughtful amendment of conventional Polyvagal sports activities sports.

One of the number one steps in adapting Polyvagal bodily video games for neurodivergence is acknowledging and respecting the character's precise neurophysiological responses. This acknowledgment turns into the cornerstone in designing wearing sports that resonate with their studies, in area of enforcing a one-duration-fits-all method.

FOR INSTANCE, the normal grounding carrying sports activities which incorporate sensory factors like touching or maintaining items, also can need modifications thinking about the sensory sensitivities traditional in neurodivergent humans. Similarly, respiration carrying sports activities, a staple in Polyvagal practices, can be tailor-made to residence the character's comfort and functionality, ensuring they may be conducive in choice to overwhelming.

Creating a supportive surroundings is paramount. It's now not sincerely about the bodily placing, but additionally approximately the relationships and interactions that inhabit that place. Establishing believe, ensuring consent, and selling autonomy are pillars in developing a supportive atmosphere for engaging in Polyvagal sporting sports.

Collaboration with multidisciplinary organizations can similarly beautify the model method. Engaging occupational therapists, speech and language therapists, and special specialists who are often part of the useful resource network for neurodivergent individuals, can provide beneficial insights. Their expertise can assist in extraordinary-tuning the carrying sports to be greater aligned with the character's needs and capacities.

Moreover, the involvement of the neurodivergent people in the variation approach is crucial. Their insights, studies, and remarks are essential in growing a model that is absolutely inclusive and powerful. This participatory technique not handiest complements the efficacy of the sports activities however moreover honors the autonomy and the lived memories of neurodivergent human beings.

Educational belongings and training for practitioners, caregivers, and the individuals themselves, is some other layer in fostering a greater nuanced know-how and effective software of Polyvagal carrying sports within the neurodivergent community. The information transfer empowers all concerned, selling a way of life of appreciate, knowledge, and shared increase.

Chapter 3: The Control Center

COMPONENTS OF THE AUTONOMIC NERVOUS SYSTEM

As we step into the area of the autonomic apprehensive device (ANS), we unveil a complicated however stylish network that silently orchestrates our interactions with the arena round us. The ANS is like an unseen conductor, critical the physiological responses that accompany our each emotion, idea, and notion. It's our frame's manipulate center for unconscious capabilities, seamlessly integrating various organs and systems to preserve a state of inner equilibrium, or homeostasis.

The ANS is extensively labeled into foremost divisions: the sympathetic and parasympathetic disturbing systems. These dual forces art work in a sensitive balance, frequently described as a dance, to control our body's responses to the myriad stimuli it encounters.

The Sympathetic Nervous System (SNS) is often dubbed the "combat or flight" device, a moniker that encapsulates its position in getting prepared our frame to reply to perceived threats. When activated, the SNS propels a cascade of reactions - accelerating the coronary coronary heart fee, dilating the students, and redirecting blood go together with the drift to the muscle mass, making organized us for movement. It's our body's accelerator, gearing us up to face annoying conditions head-on.

Conversely, the Parasympathetic Nervous System (PNS) is often associated with "rest and digest" or "feed and breed" competencies. It's the calming pressure, urging the frame to hold electricity, gradual the heart price, and beautify digestive techniques. When the tumult subsides, it's far the PNS that publications us yet again to a kingdom of calm, promoting recuperation, recovery, and boom.

At the juncture of those lies the Enteric Nervous System (ENS), frequently known as the "2nd thoughts." Residing within the gut, the ENS governs digestive methods autonomously but moreover communicates with the important frightened device, reflecting the profound interconnectivity of our body's systems.

The beauty of the ANS lies in its functionality to generally adapt to the ever-converting panorama of inner and outside demands. Each division has its precise neurotransmitters and receptors, intricately modulating responses to hold homeostasis. The dance the diverse sympathetic and parasympathetic frightened structures is not a rigid choreography but a fluid, responsive exchange, making sure we are aptly prepared to navigate the vicissitudes of existence.

Additionally, a nuanced knowledge of the ANS lays a rich foundation for exploring person variations. Neurological variations, as visible in neurodivergent people, also can have an impact on the stability and responsiveness of the ANS, supplying a compelling lens via which to check the interaction among neurodivergence and autonomic function.

Delving into the components of the ANS no longer great unveils the sophistication with which our bodies navigate the world but additionally opens avenues for appreciating the sort of human revel in. Through this lens, we are able to discover how modulation of autonomic responses can resource a spectrum of neurological evaluations, fostering a greater inclusive and compassionate know-how of the myriad strategies wherein we've interplay with the sector round us.

As we transition into the following sections, we are capable of find out how the principles of the autonomic nervous machine amplify beyond body form, serving as a metaphor for our interactions, relationships, and collective societal dynamics.

HOW YOUR BODY RESPONDS TO STRESS

The voyage into information how the frame responds to strain is akin to starting a ebook full of complex, interconnected narratives. At the middle of these narratives lies the autonomic stressful system (ANS), our organic maestro that orchestrates responses to the ever-converting outside and internal stimuli. The dynamics of pressure reaction are a nuanced interplay of severa systems, with the ANS engaging in the physiological orchestra.

When stress knocks on the door, the sympathetic concerned system (SNS) is the first to answer. It raises the alarm, catapulting the frame right proper right into a country of immoderate alert. The heart races, the breath hastens, and muscle agencies annoying up, prepared to stand the mission or flee to protection. This immediate response is a survival mechanism honed via evolution, allowing us to react hastily within the face of risk.

However, no longer all stressors are life-threatening, but our body frequently reacts as although they were. The continual activation of the SNS in reaction to regular stresses of current existence ought to have deleterious outcomes on our fitness. Over time, it may result in a kingdom of continual infection, this is frequently related to a plethora of fitness issues alongside aspect coronary coronary heart disorder, diabetes, and intellectual fitness troubles.

On the flip problem, the parasympathetic frightened device (PNS) promotes a rustic of calm, facilitating the frame's go back to a kingdom of rest and repair positioned up-strain. It's like a chilled balm, supporting to decrease the coronary coronary heart rate, ease the breath, and promote digestion. The PNS allows to repair balance, making sure that the body has a threat to heal and rejuvenate.

The dance the various SNS and PNS is a sensitive one, a harmonious balance that is critical for our wellknown health and resilience. However, this balance can be disrupted through the usage of prolonged publicity to strain, major to a rustic of autonomic imbalance. The body's capability to move returned to a country of rest and restore turns into compromised, paving the manner for chronic health problems.

Furthermore, the enteric worried device (ENS), frequently called the body's "2d mind," moreover performs a critical function within the pressure response. Situated in the intestine, the ENS communicates with the mind, influencing our mood and stress levels. The bidirectional verbal exchange some of the gut and the thoughts, known as the gut-thoughts axis, elucidates how our digestive gadget and dietary behavior can effect our pressure ranges and not unusual mood.

Understanding the body's reaction to pressure unveils the tricky tapestry of connections among our mind, frame, and the external global. It offers us the gadget to discover the profound effect of strain on our fitness, presenting a pathway toward fostering resilience and nurturing a country of balance and harmony internal ourselves.

As we traverse similarly into the realms of autonomic law and pressure, the significance of self-recognition, self-compassion, and holistic methods to managing stress grow to be apparent. This understanding empowers us to take proactive steps towards nurturing our popular health and navigating the tumultuous seas of existence with grace and resilience.

HOW YOUR BODY FINDS CALM

In the hustle of contemporary dwelling, finding calm amidst the typhoon of stressors is just like discovering an oasis in a barren region. Central to this assignment is the autonomic hectic device (ANS), a within the again of-the-scenes maestro orchestrating the frame's capacity to discover, maintain, and skip decrease lower back to a state of equilibrium. The dance of preserving calm is a choreography involving numerous components of the ANS, mainly the parasympathetic worried gadget (PNS).

When pressure retreats, the parasympathetic involved gadget steps onto the extent, offering a relaxing melody to the frame's harassed notes. It acts similar to a seasoned gardener, nurturing the frame once more to a rustic of calm, selling recuperation and rejuvenation. The PNS encourages the coronary heart fee to slow, the breath to deepen, and the muscle mass to lighten up, heralding a go back to homeostasis.

However, the direction to tranquility isn't a trustworthy one. Our frame's functionality to transition from a nation of alertness to calmness can be hampered thru persistent stressors, way of lifestyles alternatives, or maybe our very own thoughts. The cutting-edge way of life regularly places us in a continual country of arousal, wherein the symphony of calm orchestrated with the useful resource of way of the PNS is drowned out thru the cacophony of each day stressors.

Furthermore, the enteric apprehensive device (ENS), a complicated network of neurons living within the gut, moreover performs a crucial feature in our quest for calm. The speak a number of the intestine and the mind, referred to as the gut-mind axis, reflects a dating in which our digestive fitness can have an effect on our highbrow nation and vice versa. This bidirectional verbal exchange is a sworn declaration to the frame's quest for balance, wherein the dominion of our intestine can echo through the geographical regions of our emotional and intellectual well-being.

The vagus nerve, a key participant in the narrative of calm, acts as a bi-directional motorway transmitting indicators a number of the mind and the intestine. Its position in activating the PNS showcases the interconnected dance among numerous structures in conducting a kingdom of calm. By facts and nurturing the vagus nerve, humans can unlock doors to superior tranquility and resilience in opposition to strain.

The pathway to calm moreover meanders thru the location of mindfulness and rest techniques. Practices which include meditation, deep respiration, and yoga provide a haven for the overstimulated mind and frame. Through the ones practices, humans can foster a country of interest and present-centeredness, allowing a nurturing surroundings for the PNS to thrive.

RECOGNIZING AUTONOMIC RESPONSES

The autonomic worried device (ANS) operates just like an unseen conductor, orchestrating an complicated ballet of physiological responses to the rhythm of our environment, emotions, and reviews. Within this grand normal performance, recognizing the cues and cadence of our autonomic responses will become a cornerstone of self-recognition and, in the long run, self-law.

The ANS bifurcates into the sympathetic and parasympathetic worried systems, each with wonderful but complementary roles. The former springs into motion when we're going through stressors, mobilizing the frame's resources to answer to the undertaking to hand. On the alternative side, the parasympathetic annoying device is our built-in pacifier, selling relaxation and healing as soon as the typhoon has exceeded.

Recognizing the shift among those states is comparable to discerning the changing pace in a musical piece. It necessitates a tuned cognizance of the bodily, emotional, and cognitive cues that bring within the sway amongst arousal and rest.

Physical cues are possibly the most tangible signs and symptoms and signs of our autonomic responses. The quickening pulse, the shallow breath, the tensed muscle tissues—all signposts of the sympathetic electricity. Conversely, the benefit of a deep breath, the softening anxiety in our muscle mass, and the gentle rhythm of a relaxed heartbeat are the hallmarks of parasympathetic activation.

On the emotional the front, emotions of anxiety, contamination, or restlessness regularly accompany sympathetic arousal. In evaluation, a experience of calm, safety, and contentment usually deliver inside the soothing touch of the parasympathetic worried system.

Cognitively, our belief styles and mental cognizance shift with the tides of autonomic activation. Stress might also narrow our recognition, polishing our mind's lens on the perceived hazard or assignment. In a country of rest, our highbrow vista expands, deliberating a broader attitude and reflective wondering.

Moreover, the interaction among our autonomic responses and our belief of manage over our surroundings is first rate. When we perceive manage, we often find ourselves in a parasympathetic u.S.A. Of the united states, basking within the ease of predictability. Contrastingly, a lack of manage can thrust us right into a sympathetic whirl, with our frame shape bracing for the unsure.

By nurturing an reputation of those cues and their nuanced choreography, we empower ourselves to bop in music with our autonomic ebbs and flows. It's through this dance that we unlock the door to self-regulation, embracing the general spectrum of our human revel in with grace and adaptableness.

The art of spotting our autonomic responses is a cultivated understanding, honed through the years with exercise, endurance, and a mild hobby. It's a mission into the coronary heart of our lived experience, an exploration that deepens our understanding of ourselves and enriches the high-quality of our lives.

Chapter 4: The Basics Of Self-Perception

In traversing the path to self-discovery, a vital cornerstone is the knowledge and cultivation of self-notion. This element of our internal global acts as a replicate, reflecting not in reality how we view ourselves, but how we interpret and engage with the area around us. It's the lens via which we decipher the which means that that of activities, the moves of others, and our very very very own vicinity inside the grand tapestry of existence.

Self-perception starts offevolved with attention, an inward turning of interest to examine the non-forestall glide of thoughts, emotions, and sensations that drift via our attention. This gentle commentary, untainted via judgment or the need to trade, lays the foundation for a deeper expertise of oneself.

A pivotal detail in nurturing self-notion is the cultivation of mindfulness, a exercise that anchors us within the present second, thinking about a clearer view of our internal panorama. Mindfulness permits us to stand in the attention of the typhoon of our nerve-racking lives, offering an area of calm from which we are able to observe our everyday reactions to existence's annoying conditions.

Moreover, the exercising of reflective thinking can appreciably decorate our self-notion. Reflective thinking steps past mere reaction to contemplation, wherein we sift through our research, interpreting the underlying ideals and assumptions that force our behaviors. It's a moderate inquiry into the why at the back of our moves, carving a route to deeper self-information.

Building a addiction of self-statement, paired with reflective wondering, starts offevolved to loosen the grip of automatic reactions. Over time, this exercise fosters a more responsive, in vicinity of reactive, way of enticing with lifestyles.

Furthermore, the characteristic of self-compassion can't be overstated in cultivating a wholesome self-belief. A compassionate stance in the direction of oneself creates a nurturing soil from which the seeds of self-attention and expertise can flourish.

Self-belief is not a set trait however a abilities that can be honed with staying electricity and exercise. As we delve further into this bankruptcy, we're able to explore numerous practices and views that could assist the cultivation of a keen enjoy of self-belief. This exploration is much like embarking on a voyage inside, a task complete of discovery, demanding situations, and the potential for profound transformation.

The splendor of honing self-belief lies in its ripple impact. As our facts deepens, the readability with which we view ourselves and the world round us sharpens. This clarity, in flip, cultivates a life lived with aim, resilience, and a deep sense of fulfillment.

Exercises to Enhance Self-perception

As we traverse the geographical regions of self-discovery, honing our self-perception becomes a compass guiding us via the labyrinth of our inner international. This readability in notion is not in reality a passive reflection, however a knowledge that may be cultivated thru planned exercising. In this subchapter, we are able to find out diverse wearing sports geared toward nurturing a greater nuanced self-notion.

The artwork of Mindfulness Meditation offers a sturdy foundation for this agency. By anchoring our interest to the triumphing second, be it the breath, bodily sensations, or the sounds round us, we educate the thoughts to check without attachment or aversion. This practice of non-judgmental announcement regularly unveils the habitual sorts of idea and response that colour our self-belief, bearing in thoughts a greater unfiltered view of our internal workings.

Another valuable exercising is Journaling. The act of penning down our mind, emotions, and reactions to each day activities offers a reflect to have a look at the contours of our internal landscape. Over time, due to the truth the pages fill, styles start to emerge, imparting insights into our triggers, our reactions, and the huge form of emotions coloring our belief of self and others.

Engaging in Reflective Dialogue with a depended on pal or a mentor also can considerably enhance our self-notion. Through the lens of each different's compassionate reflected photo, we frequently trap glimpses of those blind spots in our self-belief that may have remained elusive otherwise.

Guided Imagery bodily sports also provide a pathway into the depths of our self-notion. Through the gentle guidance of snap shots and visualization, we are able to explore the subterranean chambers of our psyche, unearthing ideals and attitudes that form our notion of self.

In addition, practices like Mindful Walking, in which one immerses inside the full revel in of walking, feeling every nuance of motion, can shift our normal mode of autopilot to a more attentive and perceptive stance.

Each of those sports activities affords a very specific street to deepen our self-perception. Yet, the essence of this assignment remains consistent—cultivating a place of quiet observation to mild up the pathways of our thoughts. This slight illumination step by step sharpens our self-belief, paving the manner for a extra aware engagement with ourselves and the vicinity round us.

As we delve deeper into this monetary catastrophe, we will in addition find out the interplay among those carrying sports and our evolving self-perception. The voyage inward may additionally require persistence and persistence, but the treasures of insight and clarity looking ahead to us are well genuinely properly really worth the corporation.

In this realm of exploration, each step taken in enhancing self-notion is a step toward a greater actual, information, and compassionate engagement with the tapestry of lifestyles. Through the bodily sports activities elucidated proper right here, we begin to song into the symphony of our inner worldwide, each have a look at revealing any other element of our complicated, lovable self.

Recognizing Your Body's Signals

In the unfolding narrative of self-discovery, tuning into the alerts our body sends us is similar to studying a new language. This language of sensations and inner nudges is regularly diffused, yet it holds profound insights into our emotional and intellectual united states. As we project deeper into the arena of self-perception, recognizing and know-how our body's indicators turns into a cornerstone of this exploration.

The frame, a wellspring of know-how, communicates constantly. Every emotion we revel in has a physical counterpart, whether or not or not it's far the quickened heartbeat of delight, the knotted belly of tension, or the cushty shoulders of contentment. However, the cacophony of each day life frequently drowns the ones signals, leaving us disconnected from this intrinsic guidance.

One method to foster this connection is thru Mindful Sensation Awareness. By placing apart moments in our day to sit down quietly and test our frame for sensations, we begin to gather a lexicon of our body's language. This workout isn't always approximately analysis or judgment; it's about commentary and acknowledgment. Over time, spotting the interplay amongst our emotional states and their bodily expressions becomes second nature.

Another effective exercise is Breath Awareness. The breath, a barometer of our internal usa, may be every a sign and a device. Observing the breath in moments of calm in addition to in misery can provide treasured insights into our emotional global. Moreover, the usage of breath manipulate techniques also can characteristic a way to navigate through emotional waters, offering a semblance of manage in the tumult of feelings.

The exercising of Yoga and Tai Chi, each steeped in ancient knowledge, additionally provide pathways to attune to our body's signs. Through moderate movement and the cultivation of consciousness, these practices foster a deeper communicate a number of the mind and the body, thinking about a extra nuanced knowledge of our internal panorama.

Engaging in those practices diligently over time can shift our perspective, from viewing the frame sincerely as a vessel to recognizing it as a compass, supplying course within the complex terrain of self-discovery. As we develop extra adept at interpreting the signs and symptoms our body sends us, a richer statistics of our emotional and highbrow panorama unfolds. This more suitable self-perception is similar to having a talk with oneself, a verbal exchange that holds the promise of deeper insights and a extra harmonious existence.

Tracking Changes in Your Nervous System

The voyage into self-belief is similar to navigating through a dense, but enchanting wooded vicinity. As you traverse deeper, you begin to stumble upon the subtle, frequently unnoticed whispers of your body, your inner environment. One of the large elements of this internal surroundings is your apprehensive tool, an advanced network that continually communicates the usa of your internal and external surroundings. It's thru knowledge the dialect of this tool, you start to draw close to the essence of self-notion.

The apprehensive device operates just like a finely tuned orchestra, sending and receiving signals that orchestrate your interaction with the sector. It's a dynamic dance of electrical and chemical messages that continues you in music with the rhythm of lifestyles. However, the melody can from time to time turn out to be discordant, maximum crucial to states of hysteria, restlessness, or dis-ease. It's right right here, in those dissonant notes, wherein the journey of self-notion starts offevolved offevolved offevolved to deepen.

One of the profound strategies to engage on this exploration is thru Mindful Awareness, a workout that encourages a harmonious relationship amongst your thoughts and body. By adopting a stance of curious statement, you come to be attuned to the subtleties of your concerned machine. The flutter on your chest, the warmth to your palms, the chill of your breath, all emerge as messengers of your inner united states.

Additionally, practices which include meditation and somatic experiencing provide a framework to delve deeper into this communicate alongside facet your aggravating gadget. They provide a vicinity to now not truly observe but to have interaction with these signs, to apprehend their language, and to reply in a way that fosters concord and data.

Biofeedback further extends this communicate through presenting a platform to check the modifications in your frightened device in real-time. It's like having a reflect that reflects the inner shifts interior, supplying insights that have been previously obscured.

As you domesticate this practice of tracking the adjustments for your worried machine, you begin to get to the bottom of layers of self-perception. It turns into a dance of interest, wherein each step brings you in the direction of a harmonious existence. This dance is not choreographed; rather, it unfolds with each 2d, with every breath. It's an exploration that illuminates the direction of self-discovery, imparting a deeper understanding of your being.

It's essential to well known that this exploration isn't always a holiday spot but a chronic method. Each day offers a modern day opportunity to engage collectively together with your fearful tool, to recognize its indicators and to reply with focus and kindness. It's a workout that fosters a profound experience of reference to your inner worldwide, nurturing a courting that's grounded in knowledge and compassion.

INTEGRATING SELF-PERCEPTION INTO DAILY LIFE

As we navigate the voyage of self-discovery, integrating self-perception into our each day habitual emerges as a cornerstone for fostering a mindful life. This integration isn't about an intensive exchange, however a gentle incorporation of reputation into the quotidian rhythm of life. The purpose is to bridge the gap among the exploration of self-notion and the practicalities of every day living.

Self-perception isn't a passive occurrence; it is an energetic enterprise that nudges us to have interaction with our inner international even amidst the hustle of existence. The practice starts offevolved with an invitation, an invite to slow down, to pause, and to tune into the whispers of our frame and the murmurs of our thoughts and feelings.

One manner to weave self-perception into the cloth of every day life is through Mindful Pauses. These are small islands of stillness amidst the sea of every day sports activities. It can be a second of stillness before beginning the auto, a deep breath before answering a cellphone name, or a short grounding exercising earlier than entering into a meeting. These pauses act as gentle reminders, bringing us again to the prevailing second, lower back to ourselves.

Furthermore, the cultivation of a Responsive, in place of a Reactive, thoughts-set inside the course of existence contributes to this integration. It's about growing a vicinity among stimulus and response, a place wherein self-perception publications our actions. This isn't about suppression, however approximately knowledge and responding from an area of readability and compassion.

Chapter 5: Creating Your Personal Polyvagal Map

INITIAL STEPS TO CRAFTING YOUR MAP

Crafting a non-public Polyvagal Map is much like setting a sail on a voyage towards facts one's internal landscape. The Polyvagal Theory, propounded through using Dr. Stephen Porges, offers a lens to gaze into the nuances of our demanding tool, specifically the way it navigates the seas of protection and threat. Your Polyvagal Map is a custom designed compass, assisting in discerning the diffused shifts in your inner milieu, and guiding on the way to navigate via them. Here are the preliminary steps closer to crafting this insightful map.

Educating Yourself: The outset of crafting your Polyvagal Map is steeping oneself in the fundamental information of the Polyvagal Theory. Delve into dependable resources, books, or workshops that dispose of darkness from the functioning of the vagus nerve, its branches, and the way it orchestrates our responses to the environment.

Observation: Begin with a gentle announcement of your frame's responses. When do you enjoy comfortable? When do you revel in uneasy? What are the triggers that shift you from a rustic of social engagement to a kingdom of combat-or-flight or possibly freeze? These observations are the contours of your map.

Documentation: As you take a look at, report your research. You might also need to hold a every day log, jotting down the shifts in your physical sensations, emotions, and mind. This documentation will function the raw statistics to your map.

Seeking Professional Guidance: Engage with a expert who's conversant with the Polyvagal Theory. They can manual you in decoding your observations, discerning patterns, and plotting them on your map.

Reflection: Dedicate time for reflected photograph. Look at the records you've gathered, and with the steering of a professional, begin discerning patterns. Reflection lets in in information the rhythm of your irritating device and the manner it interacts along with your surroundings.

Experimentation: Based for your reflections, take a look at with particular practices like respiration carrying activities, mindfulness, or yoga to have a study how they effect your concerned device. Experimentation is ready locating what permits in guidance within the path of a country of social engagement and simplicity.

Iteration: Crafting your Polyvagal Map is an iterative approach. As you bought extra insights, refine your map. The more nuanced your map turns into, the extra it may serve as a reliable compass in navigating your inner worldwide.

Community Engagement: Share your method and observe from others who're on a comparable voyage. Community engagement offers a platform for shared mastering and help.

Creating your Personal Polyvagal Map is not a dash however a marathon. It's a slight, ongoing manner that deepens your connection in your inner worldwide, providing insights that may be lifestyles-changing. The act of crafting this map is in itself a voyage of self-discovery, one that brings you closer to expertise the language of your body and ultimately, fostering a harmonious dating with oneself.

The act of crafting your Polyvagal Map is a profound company, one which holds the capability to light up the frequently difficult to understand speak among your body and thoughts. Here, we delve deeper into the intricacies of every step to help you embark in this enlightening enterprise with a properly-primarily based footing.

Educating Yourself:

Understanding the Polyvagal Theory isn't in reality an highbrow exercising, it's an invite to the bright narrative of your apprehensive device. By exploring the underpinnings of this concept, you are taking step one within the course of growing a profound communicate together with your frame. As you take a look at the vagus nerve's position in orchestrating your responses to diverse stimuli, you can begin to take a look at the diffused whispers of your private body. Resources collectively with "The Polyvagal Theory: Neurophysiological Foundations of Emotions, Attachment, Communication, and Self-regulation" via way of Dr. Stephen Porges, can offer a sturdy foundation for your exploration.

Observation:

Observation is about fostering a compassionate hobby towards your body's responses. It's approximately noticing with out judgment. During this section, you can begin to be conscious how effective environments, interactions, or possibly reminiscences evoke specific responses for your frame. The greater you test, the greater nuanced your information becomes of the way your apprehensive tool navigates thru the waves of safety and chance.

Documentation:

This step is prepared growing a tangible mirrored picture of your observations. Your documentation must encompass now not only the bodily sensations and emotional shifts but also the out of doors occasions surrounding these shifts. Over time, this documentation will paint a photo of your tense gadget's dance with the arena spherical you.

Seeking Professional Guidance:

Engaging with a expert can offer valuable insights into decoding your observations. A professional manual can help tease out patterns, provide alternative views, and advise in addition avenues for exploration.

They can also offer guide as you navigate via the now and again turbulent waters of self-discovery.

Reflection:

Reflecting isn't a passive act but an active engagement along side your observations and documentation. It's approximately searching out patterns, making connections, and fostering a deeper know-how. Reflection can offer the gap to assimilate your studying, and at instances, unveil surprising insights approximately your anxious machine's choreography.

Experimentation:

Experimentation is the playground of discovery. It's about exploring specific practices and noticing their impact for your fearful system. Whether it's mindfulness, grounding wearing activities, or accomplishing nurturing social interactions, every check brings a present day day layer of knowledge on your Polyvagal Map.

Iteration:

Your Polyvagal Map is a dwelling, evolving entity. Each generation refines the map, making it a more accurate meditated photograph of your internal panorama. The manner of latest launch is likewise a testomony for your developing data and the dynamic communicate between you and your concerned device.

Community Engagement:

Engaging with a community of like-minded explorers can be both validating and enriching. Sharing your approach, listening to others' research, and receiving guide can significantly decorate your voyage of crafting your Polyvagal Map.

Crafting your Polyvagal Map is a profound voyage within the path of fostering a deeper, more harmonious courting together with your internal global. As you traverse thru every step, you're now not surely crafting a map, but nurturing a lifelong speak with the essence of who you're.

PRACTICAL GUIDE TO NAVIGATE YOUR EMOTIONS

Navigating the labyrinth of feelings is similar to embarking on a voyage into the unknown. The mystique of our emotional panorama regularly holds reflections of our personal fears, goals, and the innate human want for connection. The manual to guidance thru this hard community lies in information the interaction among the Polyvagal Theory and our emotional responses. This interplay acts as a compass, supporting to decode the language of our body and mind.

Tuning into the Vagal Responses:

Your voyage starts offevolved with tuning into the vagal responses. The diffused cues from your vagus nerve, the sentinel of your emotional realm, preserve vital statistics. As you start paying attention to those cues, a sample starts offevolved to spread, revealing the rhythm of your emotional ebb and go together with the go with the flow. Observing how your frame responds to emotions, whether or no longer it's a tightening in the chest with anxiety or a heat flush of happiness, is the number one stride in the path of developing a lexicon on your emotional speak.

Mindful Observation:

Mindfulness is similar to maintaining a mild, non-judgmental replicate for your emotional responses. It's approximately watching with out the urge to label or exchange. As you domesticate this dependancy of conscious remark, the nuances of your feelings begin to floor. Over time, this exercise can foster a deeper records and reputation of your emotional narrative.

Expressive Outlets:

Having expressive shops acts like vents, permitting your emotions to waft freely. Whether it is via artwork, writing, or speaking, expression creates a conduit for feelings. By undertaking expressive sports activities sports, you offer a strong passage for feelings, decreasing the probability of them becoming trapped inner.

The Practice of Self-Compassion:

Self-compassion is the gentle whisper amidst the clamor of self-judgment. It's approximately keeping area to your emotions, letting them exist without the want for validation or exchange. As you exercising self-compassion, you create a nurturing surroundings to your emotions to be explored and understood.

Connecting with Others:

Human connections act as anchors within the turbulent seas of emotions. By connecting with others, sharing reviews, and in search of resource, you create a network of harbors to are looking for safe haven at some point of emotional storms.

Educating Yourself:

Furthering your expertise approximately feelings via analyzing, attending workshops, or engaging with specialists can demystify the complexities of your emotional panorama. Knowledge is empowering; it offers the equipment crucial to navigate thru the emotional terrain with a revel in of organisation.

Seeking Professional Guidance:

Sometimes, the emotional waters may be too turbulent to navigate by myself. Seeking steerage from a expert can provide a sparkling mindset, aid, and techniques to navigate through tough emotional landscapes.

Creating an Emotional Response Plan:

Having a plan in location for responding to intense emotional reviews may be useful. This may additionally need to consist of breathing physical video video games, grounding strategies, or a list of people to the touch even as in need. Preparation gives a revel in of control, even though the emotional waves are excessive.

Understanding Emotional Triggers:

A crucial a part of navigating your emotions consists of identifying and statistics your triggers. These are out of doors or internal stimuli that might evoke robust emotional reactions. Being aware of your triggers, their origins, and their impact in your conduct is essential for cultivating a better emotional information.

Emotional Regulation Techniques:

Learning and working in the direction of emotional law techniques together with deep respiratory, mindfulness meditation, and progressive muscle relaxation can be very useful. These techniques can help you live balanced and calm, specifically in emotionally charged situations. The extra you workout, the higher you emerge as at coping with your feelings in a wholesome way.

The Role of Nutrition and Physical Activity:

Your physical health plays a large characteristic on your emotional properly-being. Eating a balanced weight loss plan and appealing in normal bodily hobby can appreciably impact your mood and energy levels. It's profitable to discover the connection among your way of existence options and your emotional u . S . A ..

Sleep Quality:

Sleep has a profound effect to your emotional stability. Ensuring you get enough restorative sleep is vital for emotional properly-being. Establishing a steady sleep time table and developing a restful environment can significantly gain your emotional health.

Understanding the Interplay of Neurotransmitters:

The polyvagal concept enables to understand how neurotransmitters, chemical compounds in our mind, have an impact on our emotional responses. Acquiring knowledge approximately the characteristic of neurotransmitters like serotonin, dopamine, and others can offer insights into handling temper swings and fostering emotional stability.

The Practice of Gratitude:

Cultivating a exercise of gratitude can significantly shift your emotional landscape. By acknowledging and appreciating the good on your lifestyles, you can foster excellent emotions and mitigate the intensity of terrible feelings.

Building Resilience:

Resilience is the functionality to get higher from adversity. Developing resilience can be finished via severa way together with keeping a terrific outlook, having strong social help, and being adaptable to alternate. The adventure in the direction of constructing resilience often outcomes in greater exceptional emotional insight and a stronger sense of self.

Creating a Supportive Environment:

Surrounding yourself with supportive and knowledge people can provide a sizeable emotional buffer. Engaging in groups or agencies that proportion your values and pastimes can foster a revel in of belonging, which in turn, can be pretty nurturing for your emotional properly-being.

Continuous Learning and Growth:

Emotional navigation is not a holiday spot however a continuous approach of mastering and boom. It's approximately evolving your knowledge, adapting to new insights, and staying open to the myriad of emotional evaluations existence has to provide.

This whole approach within the route of navigating your feelings via the lens of the Polyvagal Theory now not great enriches your emotional existence but additionally fortifies your relationships with others. It's a profound voyage of self-discovery, packed with demanding situations, learnings, and in the long run, a deeper connection with your very personal internal worldwide and the arena spherical you.

STRATEGIES FOR ADDRESSING DAILY CHALLENGES

In the search for self-interest and internal tranquility, crafting your non-public Polyvagal map is a significant stride. However, the path might not prevent right here; it's an ongoing project. Life throws severa disturbing situations our manner each day. Our potential to navigate through the each day hurdles with resilience and attraction is a actual testament to our self-discovery adventure. In this subchapter, we find out the strategies which can assist deal with each day annoying conditions using the information and equipment received to date.

A important method is making use of the Polyvagal Theory to recognize and regulate our physiological responses to strain. This includes recognizing the frame's cues and responses to numerous stressors. By knowledge the connection amongst our visceral tales and emotional responses, we're able to better manipulate our reactions to every day traumatic situations.

Moreover, cultivating an thoughts-set of mindfulness forms a cornerstone in addressing each day challenges. Mindfulness, the exercising of being present in the 2nd, can assist in searching our reactions to traumatic situations without judgment. It's approximately acknowledging our feelings and feelings without being overwhelmed thru them.

Furthermore, the exercising of grounding techniques may be instrumental. Grounding enables to supply us again to the triumphing moment, in particular at the same time as we discover ourselves out of vicinity within the whirlpool of tension or overthinking. Techniques together with focused respiration, sensory awareness, or perhaps clean physical sports like strolling or stretching may be immensely beneficial.

Daily worrying situations regularly reason an array of feelings inside us. It's vital to have an emotional outlet to specific these feelings. Engaging in sports that resonate with our inner selves, like portray, writing, or perhaps speaking to a relied on accomplice, can offer the wanted outlet.

Moreover, preserving a based each day ordinary can result in a sense of balance and predictability amidst the chaos of everyday disturbing conditions. A set up normal need to include a balanced weight loss plan, normal exercising, and suited sufficient sleep, which shape the bedrock of physical wellbeing and, by means of way of way of extension, emotional balance.

Additionally, fostering a resource machine of information and empathetic human beings can provide a protection net in the course of turbulent instances. Human connections are useful; having a supportive community can appreciably cushion the effect of each day worrying situations.

Lastly, embracing a lifelong learning thoughts-set is imperative. Every venture gives a getting to know opportunity. By adopting a curious and open mind-set, we're capable of extract precious schooling from our each day encounters and constantly evolve in our self-discovery voyage.

Through the amalgamation of these strategies, the each day disturbing situations metamorphose from being overwhelming hurdles to becoming stepping stones in the course of self-boom and inner concord. This transition is not immediately however is a slow way, regularly entire of trials, errors, and large getting to know. It's about growing a harmonious dance among our internal worldwide and the external stressful situations, leading to a fulfilling and resilient existence.

Self-Compassion:

Cultivating self-compassion is vital. It's about acknowledging that we are sure to come upon americaand downs, and it's okay.

Extending kindness and understanding in the route of ourselves within the course of hard instances can extensively alleviate the burden of challenges.

Healthy Boundaries:

Establishing healthy obstacles is an invaluable method. This involves spotting what is within our manipulate and what isn't, and reading to mention no while essential. By doing so, we shield ourselves from undue strain and keep our emotional equilibrium.

Creative Expression:

Engaging in revolutionary endeavors can be a cathartic enjoy. Whether it's thru track, art work, or writing, expressing ourselves creatively can offer an outlet for the myriad emotions evoked via using the usage of each day traumatic conditions.

Physical Activity:

Regular physical interest is a showed strain-reliever. Whether it's a brisk stroll, a run, or a yoga consultation, moving our bodies can help discharge amassed tension and foster a sense of well-being.

Mindful Communication:

Honing our conversation competencies, mainly in expressing our wishes, feelings, and obstacles, is important. Mindful conversation fosters records and collaboration, making it much less tough to navigate through annoying situations.

Time Management:

Effective time manage can drastically lessen each day strain. Prioritizing obligations, avoiding procrastination, and allocating time as it should be are abilities that may be developed with exercising.

Chapter 6: Exploring The Bond Of Mind And Body

UNDERSTANDING MIND-BODY CONNECTION

The narrative of self-exploration is one which intricately weaves the threads of the thoughts and frame right proper right into a tapestry of self-information. The thoughts-body connection isn't a completely unique idea; it's miles a profound truth that impacts each facet of our being. The interplay among our intellectual and bodily selves is a dance that shapes our perception, our reaction to the world, and our course of self-discovery. As we delve deeper into the heart of this connection, the nuances of our emotional panorama and physical sensations emerge as obvious, guiding us within the direction of a greater harmonious existence.

This symbiotic relationship among the thoughts and frame is an ode to the wonder of human existence. Our thoughts and feelings aren't surely fleeting moments of awareness; they ripple thru our physical being, manifesting as sensations, muscle anxiety, or perhaps a flutter in the chest. Conversely, our physical reviews regularly reverberate within the thoughts, evoking emotions or triggering recollections.

One of the pivotal realizations in exploring this connection is understanding that our body isn't simply a vessel for the mind, but a partner in the talk of self-exploration. The frame speaks a language of its very own, a dialect of sensations that narrates our emotional and intellectual united states. Tuning into this narrative, we start to decipher the subtle but profound messages our body conveys.

The exercise of mindfulness serves as a bridge to this statistics. It invitations us to take a seat with our reviews, to respire via the sensations, and to navigate the waters of our mind with the compass of our frame. As we attune to the rhythm of our breath, the tension in our muscle tissue, or the posture we keep, we aren't actually listening to the frame; we are carrying out a verbal exchange with our inner self.

Moreover, the Polyvagal Theory elucidates the physiological pathways that underpin this communicate. By exploring the dynamics of the vagus nerve and its characteristic in our emotional and physiological responses, we garner a deeper appreciation of the thoughts-body symphony.

A profound layer to this exploration is the belief that recovery is a holistic undertaking. Our intellectual wellness is intertwined with our physical health. The pathway to restoration isn't a solitary trek thru the geographical regions of the thoughts however a holistic day enjoy that honors the sanctity of the mind-body bond.

Furthermore, cultivating a nurturing environment every internally and externally substantially influences this connection. The spaces we inhabit, the relationships we nurture, and the self-compassion we foster, they all make contributions to a harmonious thoughts-frame communicate.

This voyage of statistics the mind-frame connection is a cornerstone inside the grander narrative of self-discovery. It's a task into the coronary heart of our being, unlocking doorways to self-compassion, resilience, and a profound information of our vicinity inside the tapestry of existence. Through this exploration, we are not merely spectators within the theater of our life, however lively individuals in scripting the narrative of our lifestyles.

BALANCING THOUGHT AND BODY-BASED PRACTICES

The odyssey of self-discovery leads one via a large panorama of studies, every unfolding layers of records in the direction of the tough tapestry of mind and frame. The equilibrium amongst notion and frame-primarily based practices bureaucracy a linchpin in harnessing the essence of this connection. A harmonious balance between the two augments the approach of self-exploration, unfurling a realm of insights that burgeon with every conscious step in this voyage.

Thought-primarily based absolutely practices, rooted in the boundless area of the mind, provide the soil from which the seeds of expertise and attention sprout. Practices such as pondered photograph, introspection, and cognitive-primarily based techniques offer a window into the narrative of our inner communicate. They allow a glimpse into the labyrinth of our thoughts, beliefs, and emotions, supplying a map to navigate through the meandering paths of our intellectual landscape.

On the opportunity facet of the spectrum, frame-based absolutely completely practices echo the primal language of sensations, embodying the whispers of the unspoken. Techniques like yoga, breathwork, and somatic experiencing invite us to descend from the living house of mind into the area of bodily sensations. They beckon within the route of a deeper resonance with the rhythms, pulses, and the silent narrative coursing thru the veins of our bodily existence.

The fulcrum among those practices lies within the artwork of conscious presence, a moderate weave between the geographical areas of concept and body. It's a dance of attention that flows seamlessly the various cerebral and the corporeal, every step a gesture of attunement to the whispers interior.

The stability is not about a inflexible equilibrium however a fluid concord that adapts to the ebb and float of our reviews. It's approximately cultivating a space wherein concept and frame-primarily based definitely practices speak in a dialect of harmony, each enriching the other, every illuminating the path of self-discovery with the mild of consciousness.

This balance is comparable to a river that meanders through the landscape of self, its waters nurturing the seeds of attention planted along the banks of thoughts and body. It's approximately fostering a nurturing environment wherein the talk among belief and body-based totally practices unfolds obviously, every one a reflected photograph and an extension of the alternative.

Mindfulness, the gentle manual on this exploration, invitations a compassionate witness to this communicate. It fosters a region of non-judgmental popularity, a haven in which the mind and body will have interplay in a candid conversation, each reading and growing from the alternative.

As the exploration deepens, the delineation amongst idea and body-based practices starts to blur, every one a thread within the same cloth of recognition. The dance the various two unfolds with a grace that speaks of a deeper information, a higher resonance with the essence of being.

Through the lens of this harmonious stability, the voyage of self-discovery transcends the sector of the cerebral, descends beyond the corporeal, and enters the area of the essence, wherein the narrative of self is not in reality understood however lived.

EXERCISES FOR MIND-BODY INTEGRATION

In the journey of self-discovery, cultivating a harmonious relationship a few of the thoughts and body is akin to developing a speak amongst antique buddies. They have been together for an entire life, but they regularly continue to be strangers to each different, their languages veiled in thriller. The realm of physical video games for mind-frame integration serves as a translator amongst those , allowing them to speak, apprehend, and help each different.

The mind, with its capability to suppose, test, and consider, holds the ability to each beautify or disrupt the natural go with the flow of frame's understanding. Similarly, the body, with its tangible sensations and historical, instinctive information, can every ground or deceive the mind. The physical sports designed for integrating thoughts and body motive to foster a cooperative spirit amongst them, nurturing a shared language that honors and uses the strengths of both.

Meditation is one such practice that beckons the mind to settle into the frame, to sense its rhythms, to honor its messages. Through the exercise of conscious meditation, one learns to take a look at thoughts without attachment, to sense sensations without judgment. The thoughts, in its serene united states of america, starts offevolved to pay interest the diffused whispers of the body, on the same time because the frame, felt and understood by way of the usage of the thoughts, starts offevolved to lighten up and specific itself with authenticity.

Yoga, a exercising historical in its roots, is a few one-of-a-kind pathway within the path of accomplishing this integration. Through a sequence of postures and breath manage, yoga invites a communicate among the physical and the intellectual. The postures mission the body, urging it to talk its boundaries and abilties to the thoughts. The breath, mild in its steerage, navigates the rhythm of this talk, making sure a communicate in region of a debate.

Beyond those practices, strategies like guided imagery, Tai Chi, and Qigong function bridges a number of the cerebral and corporeal geographical regions. They invite a present day interaction most of the imagery of the thoughts and the sensations of the frame, every enhancing the understanding and function of the opposite.

Furthermore, integrating simple practices in every day routine can also make a contribution to this talk. Mindful eating, in which one pays entire interest to the experience of consuming, feeling the texture, tasting the flavors, and being attentive to the body's alerts of starvation and fullness, may be a step toward know-how the body's language. Similarly, walking mindfully, feeling the earth underneath the feet, sensing the rhythm of the body because it actions thru space, may be a moderate reminder of the body's innate awareness.

DELVING DEEPER INTO MIND-BODY SYMBIOSIS

The union of thoughts and frame is not clearly a philosophical concept, however a tangible truth that manifests in every detail of our lives. This harmonious partnership holds the promise of a deeper knowledge of self, an exploration this is going past the superficial layers of attention into the essence of being. The symbiosis between thoughts and frame is a dance that has the capability to steer us into the geographical areas of profound self-popularity and holistic residing.

Mind-body symbiosis suggests a state of balanced interplay wherein neither overshadows the other. The mind, with its functionality for common revel in, assessment, and creativeness, reveals its grounding inside the frame's sensory critiques and intuitive focus. Conversely, the body's rhythmic lifestyles is enriched and directed with the aid of the mind's foresight and reflections. This balanced interaction creates a conduit for self-discovery, wherein the individual can traverse the landscapes of each highbrow and bodily geographical regions with cognizance and purpose.

The exploratory journey into this symbiosis unveils the implicit information this is residing inside the silent verbal exchange among intellectual and physical geographical areas. It's similar to mastering a brand new language - a language that has constantly been there, but awaits our hobby and deciphering. Through practices that promote this symbiosis, which consist of mindfulness, yoga, or possibly the clean act of attentive breathing, we start to dismantle the synthetic barrier that frequently exists among thoughts and body, paving the way for a greater covered life.

The beauty of delving deeper into mind-body symbiosis lies in its promise of exposing the innate functionality for healing, boom, and transformation that is residing internal. When thoughts and frame circulate in harmony, each supporting and informing the other, the man or woman is better prepared to navigate the complexities of life. The stressful conditions that once seemed insurmountable turn out to be possibilities for boom, the questions that seemed complicated find out their solutions in the silent whispers of symbiosis.

Moreover, the journey into thoughts-body symbiosis opens up vistas of know-how regarding our interplay with the out of doors international. The manner we perceive, reply to, and engage with the world around us is deeply encouraged through the extent of integration among our thoughts and frame. A symbiotic courting a number of the two allows a extra actual, responsive interplay with our surroundings, enriching now not in reality our non-public research, however moreover our relationships and contributions to the area at massive.

As we deepen our exploration, we find that the symbiosis among thoughts and body isn't a holiday spot however a continual method of discovery, adjustment, and realignment. It's a lifelong enterprise that holds the ability to beautify our pleasant of lifestyles, to foster a state of wholeness that is resilient, adaptable, and profoundly insightful.

APPLYING MIND-BODY PRINCIPLES IN DAILY LIFE

In the voyage of self-discovery, recognizing the profound interaction amongst thoughts and frame is a cornerstone. This recognition is not only a temporary perception but has realistic implications that may be covered into every day lifestyles. Applying mind-body ideas each day is corresponding to nurturing a garden in which the seeds of self-popularity and holistic residing are sown. It's approximately fostering a manner of existence that honors the symbiotic dating among the highbrow and bodily geographical areas, growing a fertile floor for self-boom, balance, and right dwelling.

The first step in the direction of making use of these requirements is cultivating a heightened attention of our very personal thoughts-frame interactions. This reputation can be nurtured via practices like mindfulness meditation, yoga, tai chi, or simply taking moments at some point of the day to track into our bodily sensations and highbrow state. It's approximately growing a kind of 'inner attentiveness' where we end up extra aware of the cues furnished with the useful resource of our frame and mind.

As this focus deepens, we're able to start to be conscious patterns. For example, how exceptional thoughts may cause bodily tension, or how physical soreness could probable cloud our highbrow clarity. Recognizing the ones styles is empowering because it lays the inspiration for greater conscious choice-making and responses to lifestyles's situations.

Chapter 7: Effective Coping Strategies

UNDERSTANDING COPING MECHANISMS

In navigating the turbulent waters of life, people often are seeking out stable haven in coping mechanisms, the personal strategies devised to control pressure, trouble, or pain. These mechanisms are like individualized shields, employed to protect in competition to or mitigate feelings and tales perceived as threatening or overwhelming. They are the body and thoughts's way of searching for to maintain equilibrium amidst the storms of life.

Coping mechanisms are born out of necessity and are original through a large extensive variety of things which consist of private opinions, temperament, and the encircling surroundings. They aren't truely an escape direction from discomfort, however a method to device, adapt, and respond to lifestyles's various circumstances.

There are numerous coping techniques human beings lean on. Some are adaptive, promoting growth and healing, even as others are maladaptive, in all likelihood stifling boom and exacerbating issues. The essence of knowledge coping mechanisms lies within the popularity in their dual nature.

Adaptive coping mechanisms collectively with problem-fixing, seeking out social guide, and the use of relaxation techniques, inspire an active engagement with traumatic conditions. They foster a experience of empowerment and control, promoting resilience and the purchase of treasured life competencies. These mechanisms don't shrink back from the difficulty available however face it head-on, searching for decision or recognition.

On the turn element, maladaptive coping mechanisms like avoidance, substance abuse, or denial, provide transient treatment on the fee of lengthy-term resolution. They should likely ease the pain momentarily however frequently bring about a vicious cycle of dependency and avoidance of the underlying troubles.

Delving into one's coping mechanisms calls for a combination of self-meditated photo, honesty, and possibly, guidance from a professional therapist. It's approximately dissecting the man or woman, characteristic, and effect of these mechanisms on one's lifestyles. This understanding sheds slight on non-public behavioral patterns, helping inside the cultivation of more adaptive techniques.

Moreover, it's crucial to hold in mind that coping mechanisms are not constant; they're malleable and can evolve over the years with aware effort and guide. Unveiling the intricacies of one's coping strategies is corresponding to unlocking a door to advanced self-cognizance and advanced existence manipulate.

As human's development in unraveling their coping mechanisms, they begin to update maladaptive strategies with extra adaptive ones. This transition isn't always a bounce however a gradual climb, requiring staying energy, dedication, and a nurturing surroundings.

Understanding coping mechanisms is corresponding to embarking on an day experience into the coronary coronary heart of one's coping worldwide, with the promise of gaining insights which have the electricity to convert existence's stressful conditions into stepping stones toward private increase and resilience.

In sum, gaining a deeper statistics of coping mechanisms is a pivotal step within the way of personal improvement. It's a challenge that not pleasant illuminates the direction to better intellectual and emotional health however moreover enriches the quality of existence. Through this know-how, people equip themselves with the gadget vital to navigate lifestyles's adversities with a reinforced feel of organization and resilience.

Chapter 8: Where Is The Vagus Nerve And What Does It Do?

Wholesome Vagus Nerve is essential to many elements of our well-being and day by day functioning. It's the throughway a number of the thoughts and the body talking to effects runs endless automated body techniques we don't be aware of, like breathing and digestion. This single nerve also continues our functionality to recover from strain and regulates our moods.

Originating from the brain stem, the Vagus Nerve travels thru the face and down each elements of the neck, branching out to hook up with most organs within the body, and ends inside the abdomen. As the tenth cranial nerve, it's the longest within the autonomic traumatic machine and has every sensory and motor capability, making it crucial in plenty of frame strategies just like those listed below.

Functions of the Vagus Nerve

Controls coronary heart charge lowers the coronary heart fee and blood pressure.

Manages muscular tissues Directs muscle actions inside the throat, voice subject, and meals passage, facilitating features like swallowing and speakme.

Handles digestion Supervises the digestive tracts operations from mouth to bowel.

Sensory features Processes data from the ear, tongue, and throat which include taking note of and tasting.

Anti-inflammatory reaction Sends a signal to different frame elements to lower infection.

Improves immunity Stimulates the immune tool.

Balances the concerned device Key in returning the involved tool to a comfortable nation after pressure.

Regulates breathing: Aids in calming respiratory patterns inside the lungs and diaphragm.

Controls worry reaction and emotional regulation: Crucial in getting better from pressure and tension and is chargeable for that "gut feeling" and "butterflies".

Produces sweat and salivation: Handles sweat production and salivary capabilities.

Speech: Assists within the manufacturing and modulation of our voice.

Sexual arousal: Plays a characteristic inside the body's responsiveness to sexual stimuli.

Regulates urination: Responsible for the muscle movement of the bladder.

Detoxification: Connects to all detoxifying organs.

When the Vagus Nerve is in pinnacle-great state of affairs, our minds and our our bodies regularly experience rejuvenated and rested; we find out ourselves greater energetic, mentally sharp, and satisfied to socialize. There's an innate experience of calm and equilibrium, making worrying conditions extra viable and pleasures greater enjoyable.

A Key Part of the "Rest and Digest" System

The body has crucial factors to its annoying system: the Central Nervous System including the mind and spinal wire, and the Peripheral Nervous System crafted from nerves that department out from the number one worried device and talk to the rest of the body. The Peripheral Nervous System consists of the Somatic Nervous System, controlling voluntary actions and the Autonomic Nervous System (ANS) which manages automated frame responses. The primary branches of the ANS are: the Sympathetic Nervous System (SNS), which facilitates us stay to inform the story even as going through strain and chance and the Parasympathetic Nervous System (PNS) which allows us to relax, heal and thrive. The Vagus Nerve makes up a whopping seventy five% of the PNS and hyperlinks the mind and spinal cord to the digestive device.

When We're Surviving

The Sympathetic Nervous System (SNS) springs into motion while we're confronted with stressors. This can variety from impending physical threat to everyday stressful conditions which includes artwork pressures, economic troubles, or emotional upsets. This "combat or flight" response is a survival mechanism, making geared up the body to each face the hazard or flee from it. When we enjoy strain, our body's essential priority shifts to addressing that instant danger, and this may make us sense annoying, nerve-racking, and hyper-alert.

Key responses added on by way of manner of the SNS include:

Heart charge will increase to pump blood extra effectively to important organs and muscle agencies.

Blood go with the flow redirects often to muscle groups, making geared up for bodily movement.

Pupils dilate, deliberating better vision in ability low-mild conditions.

Adrenaline is released to enhance power and application stages.

Digestion slows so that power is prioritized for instant response rather than prolonged-term techniques.

When We're Thriving

In reaction, the Parasympathetic Nervous System (PNS) acts because the counterbalance to the SNS. Once the right away chance or stressor has handed, the PNS desires to convey the body again to its baseline, specializing in lengthy-term nourishment, restoration, and stability while we "relaxation and digest".

Primary functions of the PNS encompass:

Heart rate decreases and stabilizes.

Digestion reactivates and promotes the digestive manner.

Muscles lighten up.

Reduces pressure hormones.

Redirects energy to hold it for destiny desires.

Keeping the Body in Balance from Stress

Balance, or homeostasis, is the body's final purpose. Regardless of the severa outside and inner elements we come upon every day, our frame continuously strives to keep a kingdom of equilibrium. This stability isn't approximately staying even though or static; rather, it's a dynamic way of subtle modifications made in actual-time, ensuring our body's structures feature optimally.

Stress, in its diverse office paintings—be it environmental, bodily, emotional, or intellectual—disrupts this equilibrium. Think of pressure as a scale tipping to one aspect.

For example, recollect moments whilst you've faced a annoying event, like narrowly keeping off a automobile twist of fate. The initial adrenaline rush—fast heartbeat, traumatic muscle tissue, and application—is a testament to the frame's Sympathetic Nervous System at paintings. However, as fast because the threat passes, it's the vagus nerve's responsibility, as a key player within the PNS, to assist deliver the body decrease back to calmness, slowing the coronary coronary heart charge, enjoyable muscle corporations, and restoring rest. This shift reduces inflammation, and units the quantity for recuperation and repair. A well-functioning vagus nerve is important for our capability to correctly control and recover from stress, ensuring our body stays in its desired state of dynamic equilibrium.

The Crossroads of Your Brain and Body

The have an impact on of the vagus nerve extends past connections with severa important organs. It acts as a conduit for 2-manner verbal exchange a number of the thoughts and body. This nerve sits at a crucial intersection, or crossroads, translating highbrow states into physiological responses and vice versa.

One instance of this is the vagus nerve's position in its involvement in the gut-mind axis, as it links our crucial fearful device (generally the mind and spinal cord) to our enteric nervous gadget (the complicated network governing our gastrointestinal tract). Gut health, as studies increasingly indicates, can considerably affect highbrow properly-being. Feelings of hysteria or depression could probably originate from, or be exacerbated through, disruptions in our intestine plants.

Similarly, our highbrow states will have an impact on intestine characteristic, explaining why a few humans would possibly enjoy stomach upsets throughout traumatic times. The vagus nerve is the number one channel facilitating this speak, making sure that the mind is up to date approximately intestine health and that the gut, in flip, responds to the thoughts's cues.

Aside from the intestine/thoughts axis, the vagus nerve vitally communicates with many systems and components of the mind and frame and is essential in ensuring that our mind and frame feature in concord. Recognizing its position underscores the significance of acknowledging that mental nicely-being is installed to bodily fitness, and vice versa.

You will discover ways to prompt the restoration electricity of this critical nerve later in this e-book to assist assist your famous nicely being.

three

Stress, Trauma and the Vagus Nerve

I

n our rapid-paced international, strain has emerge as a common denominator for hundreds. But what function does the vagus nerve play on this? Let's check how stress and trauma will have an effect on our fitness and nicely-being.

The Impact of Physical and Emotional Stress on Your Mind and Body

Stress, whether or not bodily or emotional, starts offevolved a cascade of reactions sooner or later of the frame. Let's discover the ones stressors and the sensations they elicit inner us.

Think of the immediately aftermath of a physical damage or intense workout. Muscles could probably disturbing up, coronary heart fee can increase, and respiration can also furthermore end up speedy. You may additionally revel in a rush, regularly described as an adrenaline surge. If this stress persists, fatigue sets in. The body might also ache, movements can emerge as gradual, and there's an overarching choice for relaxation and recuperation.

On the emotional the front, demanding situations like grief, administrative center pressure, or dating problems have their non-public set of affects. The mind may also moreover race with a flurry of thoughts, making awareness tough. Sleep patterns might be disrupted, most important to each insomnia or excessive sleepiness. Emotionally, feelings of sadness, irritability, or tension might dominate. Some might also moreover experience physical symptoms too: a tightness in the chest, a churning belly, or even random aches and pains without a easy physical reason.

Healthy vs Unhealthy Stress

Stress, as a physiological reaction, isn't inherently bad. In fact, our frame's capability to react to strain has been important for survival over millennia. However, it's crucial to distinguish amongst acute (short-term) stress, which may be useful, and continual (lengthy-time period) pressure, which may be detrimental to our fitness.

Acute Stress: Acute stress is a proper away reaction to right now threats, recognized frequently because the "combat or flight" reaction. This sort of stress can heighten our senses, boost our physical average performance, and sharpen our cognitive characteristic. Think of the right now reaction you'd have in case you all of sudden located a snake for your course or the stepped forward attention during a critical presentation. Once the threat or project passes, our body normally returns to its baseline usa and occasionally this strain makes us more potent, faster, smarter, etc.

Chronic Stress: Contrarily, continual strain persists over prolonged intervals with out massive remedy or rest among worrying situations. This can be because of ongoing paintings pressures, lengthy-term health issues, or extended economic issues. Such extended publicity to strain hormones and a non-prevent country of heightened alertness can bring about intense mental and physical health issues.

Impacts of Chronic Stress on Health

Mental: Leads to issues like despair, tension, and insomnia. It can exacerbate feelings of helplessness, hopelessness, and may result in emotional burnout.

Physical: Increases the chance of illnesses which include high blood stress, coronary heart disorder, diabetes, and weight troubles.

The immune gadget receives weakened, leading to frequent infections. There's additionally an improved hazard of gastrointestinal problems like Gastroesophogeal Reflux Disease (GERD), gastritis, and ulcerative colitis.

Cognitive: Impairs cognitive features main to awareness troubles, forgetfulness, and desire-making issues.

While acute pressure can be a healthful and adaptive response to instant challenges, persistent pressure, if not managed, can wreak havoc on both our intellectual and bodily well-being.

Trauma

Trauma isn't always just like pressure in that it's an emotional response to actual or perceived damage or risk, along side an twist of destiny, bullying, residing in an risky or unstable surroundings, a bodily assault, or a herbal disaster. A person can enjoy it themselves or witness it. Usually, a person may be in surprise and then denial right after the event. They may be considerably stricken by acute trauma (a single occasion) or even extra affected by chronic trauma (continual and extended trauma, along aspect abuse). Either can cause Post Traumatic Stress Disorder (PTSD).

Chapter 9: Potential Impacts Of Acute Trauma On Health

Mental: Leads to marvel and denial, anxiety, immoderate emotional reactions like fear, anger, disappointment and guilt and normal recollections of the occasion in mind, panic attacks, confusion and temper swings.

Physical: Creates sleep troubles, physical symptoms and signs like nausea, dizziness, fatigue, or muscle tension, being effects startled or jumpy, elevated coronary heart charge or palpitations, hyperventilation or shortness of breath.

Cognitive: Impairs capacity to hobby and make selections, results in reminiscence gaps, or surprising reminiscences that disrupt the present day 2d.

Behavioral: Causes avoidance, social withdrawal, and generally being on alert.

Potential Impacts of Chronic Trauma on Health

Mental: Leads to persistent tension and worry, depression, feeling numb or disconnected, creates low shallowness.

Physical: Increases in persistent fatigue regardless of sleep, digestive issues like Irritable Bowel Syndrome (IBS) or belly aches, not unusual tension or migraine headaches and unexplained continual ache like joint or muscle ache, progressed risk of coronary heart disease, PTSD, insomnia, night time time sweats or oversleeping, decrease immune tool functioning, unexplained weight benefit or loss, or sexual disease.

Cognitive: Leads to recognition, memory and preference-making problems. A character will re-enjoy the trauma, turn out to be greater inflexible of their thinking, and could have reading issues.

Behavioral: Increases avoidance of reminders of trauma, insomnia or nightmares, self-harming, substance abuse or addictive behavior.

The affects of acute or persistent trauma can variety broadly among humans. Not anybody will revel in the ones type of signs and symptoms, and some may additionally enjoy others not indexed proper right here. It's constantly critical to speak about with healthcare professionals if someone believes they're tormented by the affects of pressure or trauma that is substantially affecting them. Recognizing and addressing the signs and symptoms and signs and symptoms and symptoms of these problems is pivotal for retaining holistic health.

Polyvagal Theory

Dr. Stephen Porges' Polyvagal Theory gives a street map to statistics that the Autonomic

Nervous System and specially the Vagus Nerve, play an vital function in regulating our conduct and fitness.

Porges believes that after we're in a nation of danger, our worried system doesn't regulate our organs or control our social relationships with success and our priorities alternate. Instead of focusing on growth, health, rest, and connecting with others, we popularity on survival inside the gift. When a danger or trauma has exceeded, our our our bodies can act as even though the hazard continues to be gift and pass right into a country of prolonged strain and anxiety. We may be left with trauma that modifications the autonomic states of our our bodies, not simply in our reminiscences. Treating trauma can be greater about treating the physiological reaction than the experience itself.

Trauma or immoderate strain also can motive emotional dysregulation, on the same time as there's a mismatch between our inner reactions and the outside surroundings.

Imagine the jarring sensation of feeling immoderate panic on a quiet, normal day or the unease of being overly calm for the duration of a disaster. Key signs and symptoms include unpredictable temper swings, immoderate reactions to mild stimuli, and a steady feeling of being emotionally out of manage.

Stimulating the Vagus Nerve Taps Directly into Rest, Digest and Healing

The right charge of information the Polyvagal Theory lies in its software. The purpose is to retune and balance the stressful device to lower strain and heal that trauma thru giving it the cues of protection via direct activation of the"rest and digest" device with vagus nerve wearing sports activities. Recognizing that we're in a role to influence our automatic responses this manner, is a transformative attention. The physical video games stated on this ebook offer practical machine to promote a greater healthy Vagus Nerve. It's like schooling a muscle: the greater you stimulate your Vagus Nerve in a selected way, the stronger and further inexperienced it becomes. Regularly operating toward those wearing sports can help refine your strain responses, decorate your social interactions, and make sure that your emotional reactions are more attuned to your surroundings.

four

Healthy Vagal Tone Means a Healthy Body and Mind

V

agal tone refers to the interest and responsiveness of the vagus nerve. In easy phrases, it's a manner to gauge how nicely the vagus nerve competencies. A higher vagal tone often indicates that the nerve is running optimally, all of sudden responding to modifications and facilitating powerful conversation among the brain and body. Higher vagal tone has moreover been associated with the following:

Physical Signs

Stable coronary heart fee: Regulates coronary heart price. A ordinary, consistent coronary coronary heart rate without sudden fluctuations.

Consistent breathing styles: Smooth, deep breaths with out shortness of breath or rapid respiration.

Good digestive feature: Efficient digestion and regular bowel actions with out common disruptions or discomforts.

Healthy gag reflex: A realistic and responsive gag reflex.

Optimal blood pressure: Maintaining blood strain inside a healthful variety.

Swift recuperation after pressure: The ability to fast pass again to a non violent nation after dealing with pressure.

Anti-inflammatory: Reduced inflammatory responses in the frame, primary to fewer instances of inflammatory conditions or flare-ups.

Efficient salivation: Stimulates the manufacturing of saliva offering good enough salivation, in particular inside the route of meals..

Reduced instances of nausea or dizziness: The vagus nerve can on occasion be a issue in emotions of nausea or dizziness, so fewer episodes can recommend it's functioning well.

Normal swallowing reflex: Proper function and coordination in the course of swallowing.

Absence of continual fatigue: Feeling energized and not continuously tired or fatigued.

Healthy pores and skin: Better blood flow into, which may additionally arise as a healthful pores and pores and pores and skin complexion.

Emotional and Cognitive Signs

Emotional balance: Fewer episodes of temper swings or emotional outbursts.

Resilience to pressure: Ability to get higher from annoying sports activities extra speedy, showing adaptability.

Reduced tension: Lesser emotions of restlessness or steady worry.

Better recognition: Enhanced interest and the ability to stay on venture.

Improved memory: Efficient bear in thoughts and processing of information.

Enhanced social connection: Increased interest in social interactions, feelings of connectedness, and expertise of others' emotions.

Reduced symptoms and symptoms and signs and symptoms of despair: Lesser feelings of disappointment, hopelessness, or disinterest in previously a laugh sports activities.

Positive outlook: Tendency to view demanding situations with optimism and keep a hopeful mind-set.

Greater mindfulness & presence: Ability to stay inside the second and be absolutely engaged in the cutting-edge pastime.

Enhanced trouble-solving competencies: Ability to think extensively and discover effective solutions to disturbing situations.

Good sleep styles: Regular sleep styles and feelings of restfulness upon waking up.

Intuitive choice making: Trusting one's gut feeling and making alternatives with clarity.

Less irritability: Reduced impatience and frustration in reaction to minor inconveniences or annoying situations.

Balanced libido: Healthy hobby in sexual interest, neither hyperactive nor suppressed.

Increased empathy: Ability to understand and percent the emotions of others, promoting higher interpersonal relationships.

Reduced fear reaction: Less inclination to react with undue fear to non-threatening conditions.

Measuring Vagal Tone

Aside from symptoms and signs and symptoms of wholesome vagal tone, there's a way to degree your vagal tone not right away. Heart Rate Variability (HRV) can take a look at the performance of your vagus nerve. It measures the time variation among successive heartbeats. Generally talking, a higher variability within the time amongst heartbeats regularly shows a more healthy and additional responsive coronary heart, indicating higher vagal tone. It's like having a bicycle with 12 speeds in preference to 2, so you can extra with out trouble experience at unique speeds on a greater variety of terrain.

What is Average HRV?

For adults, HRV spans a massive variety and can be everywhere from beneath 20 to over 200 milliseconds (ms). The measurement can be very touchy and particular to absolutely everyone. Generally, your HRV will decrease with age and is a superb deal less related to your sex and health stage. A normal HRV for a youngster to twenty year vintage is fifty 5–one hundred and five ms at the same time as for those 60 and up, it's 25–45 ms. It can change hourly or every day and can be impacted with the resource of way of such things as getting proper sleep, how you're feeling, medicinal capsules, contamination, your environment, genetics, in case you're dehydrated and various factors. The remarkable thing is to diploma it based definitely for your very personal non-public averages. The score is measured at night time so there are fewer affects of the strain you address at some point of the daytime. The maximum accurate analyzing is probably on a continuous electrocardiogram, or EKG thru your medical doctor or, as of this writing, the AIO Smart Sleeve. Though in all likelihood not as correct, you can measure and spot how your HRV is trending over weeks and months on accessible wearable devices, which may be treasured records for you. They are to be had at unique rate factors and can be worn in your wrist (Fitbit, Whoop Strap), as a chest strap (Polar) or a hoop (Oura) on your finger.

Check to appearance what they're nicely ideal with and which apps can paintings with them. Popular apps that paintings with chest coronary heart rate video show devices are Elite HRV and HRV4 Training, despite the fact that they may be geared more in the direction of athletes.

While it's no longer critical to song your HRV, thru deciding on the proper tool tailor-made for your desires and rate range, you can get precious insights approximately your health as well pointers on at the same time as you can address a project or even as it's better to relaxation and get higher. Let's check the sporting sports which can decorate your Vagal Tone and assist you sense extra comfortable.

Chapter 10: 50 Quick Vagus Nerve Exercises And Practices

Chicken you're careworn and busy is while you can want these sports activities the maximum. They will help your frame and mind get out of the protecting pressure mode, assisting you loosen up via triggering your calming and recuperation country as an alternative. Most importantly, they're capable of help located you right into a greater calm nation bodily and mentally at once at the same time as now not having to think or over think about it.

These mind and body sports can artwork inside the instantaneous, brief or prolonged-time period, based totally totally mostly on the manner you observe them. If a person cuts you off at the same time as riding in website visitors and also you discover yourself irritated and your coronary heart is racing, you can at once do a respiratory exercise to calm yourself down, supplying a brief reset for your body and mind. For quick or prolonged-term outcomes, a every day exercise is usually recommended. Over time, this may deliver over into your ordinary life, so you received't have as lots of a response to common stressors.

Life may be busy—harnessing the strength of the vagus nerve doesn't must require hours of willpower. The sporting occasions in this ebook have been selected due to the reality they will be completed in only 5 minutes or much less, so even when you have a packed schedule, you can discover pockets of time to do them.

There are a massive kind of sports activities sports and practices from stretching to respiration to meditation to growing a track and more. Some are easy to do nearly everywhere you're, a few require precise poses or so that it will lie down and you may use apps or motion pictures for a few.

How to Maximize These Exercises

Before you begin any exercising, it allows to pause, loosen up and take some breaths, if viable.

If you're now not using an app or video, positioned your mobile cellphone away and flip it off.

You can growth blessings by doing some of these physical video video games concurrently, together with a respiratory workout while coloring or on foot.

The respiration bodily sports are the satisfactory for immediate results that you can do virtually everywhere. Always inhale through your nose, if possible.

If you've got greater than five minutes, you could stack those and do numerous in a row, or take breaks at a few level in the day and encompass them.

Your body likes ordinary and will reply better if you do the ones carrying sports on the same time each day,or on some shape of time table, despite the fact that that's not important.

Spending greater time (15–20 min.) on some bodily games can increase your blessings.

You apprehend your self first-rate, so ensure these are stable that allows you to do. If you feel agitated, stop the workout. I encourage you to touch a fitness professional in case you aren't certain about any of the sports activities or practices. Each humans is incredible and will respond in every other manner to precise bodily sports. You may additionally find out which you gravitate inside the direction of high-quality techniques greater than others, or that a few simply artwork better for you.

Different people have differing ranges of strain, tension, trauma, depression, contamination and intellectual and bodily responses—we are anybody. The greater immoderate your signs and symptoms and symptoms and signs and symptoms, the extra healing you will want and you may already be, or need to complement those sporting sports with distinct remedies or techniques. Often, more than one focused solutions will offer you with better results, similar to workout and eating healthy food will provide you with a more fit and additional healthful body in evaluation to exercise on its very very own.

A incredible manner to begin and forestall your day is with the useful resource of doing respiratory physical games, which you could do in bed.

Keep in mind that the crucial component to those physical sports is consistency. By integrating them into your every day everyday, in spite of the reality that only for a couple of minutes, you may start to see profound consequences through the years.

FOR GENERAL HEALTH

Slow and Deep Breathing together with your Diaphragm

Relax first. Stand, sit down down in a chair or lie down without trouble.

Inhale slowly and deeply via your nostril for a depend of four—your stomach

will upward thrust.

Pause and preserve for 4 counts.

Then exhale slowly thru pursed lips, as in case you're blowing up a balloon for a count wide variety of 8. Your belly will fall.

Repeat for 5 mins.

Tip: You can location one hand for your chest and one to your stomach. If your chest is growing and falling, you are the use of your lungs, no longer your diaphragm. If you enjoy dizzy or are yawning, you are overbreathing or trying too tough. Just allow circulate of that manipulate, relax and begin over.

Neck Stretch

Sit instantly. Put your proper hand at the top and left thing of your head, lean your head to the proper and then lightly pull your head to the right at the same time as tensing and stretching the muscle corporations at the left component of your neck. Hold for 20 seconds.

Do the same on the other component and maintain for 20 seconds.

Repeat 2-3 instances on every aspect.

Tip: Ensure your shoulders live comfortable and decreased.

three

Laughter

Think of a funny 2d, watch a humorous video, or in reality faux chortle until it

turns proper.

Variation

Laughter yoga training may be a terrific guided manner to result in laughter.

The Basic Exercise: with the aid of the use of Stanley Rosenberg

Sit or lie down and clasp your hands within the again of your head to cradle it. Your elbows could be pointing outward to the proper and left.

Keep your head coping with earlier and desk sure and in conjunction with your eyes handiest, look to the right, preserving your eyes open. Hold the location for about a minute or till you feel the need to yawn, sigh or breathe deeply.

Move your eyes once more to the center and relaxation. You might possibly need to get your bearings.

Now, flip and skip your eyes most effective to the left, all all over again keeping for approximately a minute.

Move your eyes all over again to the center and relaxation.

Tip: Try rotating your head to the left and proper earlier than you do this exercise and then attempt it after the exercise. You want to test that your head will rotate similarly.

Note: Some humans may additionally revel in greater traumatic after this exercising, especially in case your anxiety is worse if subjects are too calm and quiet. If so, please artwork thru this collectively together together with your therapist.

This exercising can assist with neck and shoulder tension, headaches or even migraines.

Trapezius Twist: via way of Stanley Rosenberg

Grab your elbows.

Rock them back and forth at your waist diploma for five seconds, your chest degree for five seconds after which, above your shoulders for 5 seconds.

Tip: Good to do when you've been sitting for a while and your head or posture is leaning in advance or in case your posture is slumping.

Mindfulness Meditation

Sit upright without problems, so that you revel in cushty.

Breathe lightly and word your inhale and exhale.

Do a body experiment and be aware how your frame feels from your feet, element by using detail all the way in your head. Feel the floor you're sitting on, the temperature of the room, the garments to your frame, and so on.

Your mind will wander and mind will come into your head. Don't fight them. Instead permit your thoughts come and skip, searching at and then releasing them. Then reputation returned on your breath. As you still exercise this, you could have fewer distractions.

Start through way of meditating for 2 minutes and artwork as a lot as five.

Tip: Ensure you're in a quiet surroundings to truly immerse within the experience. You can also use a guided meditation app or internet internet page to comply with together with.

Vagus Nerve Neck Massage

Locate your Sternocleidomastoid (SCM) muscle: look within the replicate and turn your head to the left. The diagonal muscle alongside your neck becomes more seen and runs from the top of your inner collar bone to in the back of your ear. This is what we can be massaging.

With your head grew to become, firmly pinch along the proper SCM. Lean your head all over again at the equal time as squeezing it to stretch it. Then rotate your head to the proper. Hold for approximately 30 seconds earlier than shifting to each other spot. Start lower and artwork your way as a lot as under your jaw. This want to no longer harm.

You can also experience tension in a few additives that you'll want to rub down extra.

Repeat on the other issue.

Yoga Sequence for Relaxation (amateur diploma)

Child's Pose

Begin via kneeling at the ground.

Sit decrease again onto your heels and bend ahead, laying your torso amongst your thighs.

Stretch your fingers inside the front of you and lighten up for approximately 1-2 minutes.

Legs-Up-The-Wall Pose

Transition with the aid of sitting next to a wall.

Gently swing your legs up onto the wall on the same time as lying decrease lower back onto the ground. Make certain there's a comfortable distance amongst your sitting bones and the wall.

Relax on this function for 2-three mins.

Corpse Pose

Finally, lie to your over again, flat on the ground together with your legs and arms spread quite absolutely apart.

Close your eyes and attention on deep, even breaths.

Remain in this position for approximately 1-2 minutes.

This yoga series is designed to lighten up the body and stretch key muscle organizations. It's a extremely good way to unwind and sell regular nicely-being.

Singing

Sing along to a favorite music within the vehicle or shower.

Variation

Sing in a choir or institution—just ensure there can be no strain, so that you can loosen up and function amusing.

Good for your immune device, reduces pressure, trauma, and tension. Singing with others increases your experience of belonging.

Box Breathing

Sit effects.

Inhale through your nostril for four seconds.

Hold your breath for 4 seconds.

Exhale thru your nostril for four seconds.

Hold your breath for four seconds.

Repeat 3 to five instances

Can calm you quick and beautify readability. Good for trauma, depression, tension.

Qi Gong: Shaking The Tree

Stand collectively with your feet flat on the floor, shoulder width apart, loosen up and keep close your fingers at your elements.

Tuck your butt in and in advance and straighten your again.

Relax your frame. Keeping your ft and balls of your toes on the floor, leap

up and down on on your heels. Keep your body loose from the knees up and permit it

circulate, shake or soar round. The pace and depth are your selections, however start gently.

Breathe thru your nose deep into your diaphragm.

Do this for 1 minute, then growth it to three, and then 5 mins. When you forestall, you may sense a ripple of strength on your body, like while you throw a stone in water.

Variation

You can begin through way of lightly bouncing collectively along with your feet flat at the ground and boom intensity.

Tip: This is a superb practice to do every day.

Helps with emotional regulation, releases stress, anxiety, melancholy and bad feelings, relaxes and energizes. Helps drain and purge lymph nodes.

Grounding Exercises

Walk Barefoot: Take your footwear and socks off and positioned your naked ft at the ground—on grass, sand or dust.

Variations

Lie on the Ground: This offers you extra pores and skin to earth touch—you may lie at the grass to your out of doors or at a park, or on sand on the seashore.

Go Underwater: Wade in a lake or flow, swim within the ocean.

Grounding Equipment: If you can't glide outdoor, you can placed a steel rod within the earth that is related to your body through a cord offered as a bundle. Alternatively, there are grounding mats, sheets, blankets, socks, bands and patches.

For Anxiety: Ground at the same time as you're having a panic attack.

For Insomnia: Ground with the sunrise in order to help re-set your circadian rhythm, if that's a part of the cause you are having troubles sleeping. (20 minutes of grounding is great for this).

For Depression: Ground each day. Inflammation performs a characteristic in melancholy too. Create a ordinary to be out of doors every day like gardening, nature photographs, chicken searching, reading, taking note of tune or a podcast, journaling together together along with your bare ft in the grass.

Note: Grounding is placing your frame in direct contact with the earth's electric powered fee. Electrons get finished to our our bodies which allows to decorate our blood go with the flow, destress and balance our frightened gadget.

Helps with continual fatigue, continual pain, anxiety, despair, inflammation, sleep troubles and cardiovascular contamination.

Chapter 11: Loving-Kindness Meditation

Send emotions of affection, compassion, kindness and forgiveness to yourself and others.

Follow the listing under:

Friends, family, cherished ones and friends.

People who're suffering anywhere within the international.

Someone who has assist you to down or harm you.

Forgive yourself for any damage or negativity you gave yourself or others.

Tip: If you embody those 4 organizations, it emphasizes the humanity in honestly everybody.

Increases effective feelings, compassion, emotional processing, decreases PTSD, migraines, chronic pain, and improves social bonds and bodily fitness which encompass ache manage. Helpful for despair, chronic stress and trauma.

Mindful Walking

Pay interest to the sensations of your frame and your surroundings.

Start taking walks a touch slower than normal.

Open your thoughts and your senses, noticing what is taking place from 2nd to second. What does it look, odor and sound like? How do your ft or palms enjoy? Is there a breeze, or is the solar shining on you? Be aware of your breath. You can try this everywhere you are: inside the united states, city, or nature.

If your mind wanders, gently guide it back in your breath, the walk, and what's taking location outside and inside of you.

When you're completed, be though and take more than one deep breaths.

Tip: There are extended advantages in nature.

Helps with depression and anxiety, the immune tool and highbrow rest. Opens you to a enjoy of "awe".

Listen to music

For Relaxation: Listen to music that has a smooth melody and a slow pace with out a lyrics. Best length: five-19 minutes, relying on the man or woman.

Good for reducing muscle anxiety, having fewer bad mind and snoozing higher.

Variation

To Boost your temper: Music with a using rhythm, fast pace, and superb or giant lyrics in genres like Pop, Rock, Classical and Hip Hop. Best duration: five-14 minutes, relying at the man or woman.

Tip: During workout, being attentive to song can help a faster healing afterwards.

Good for having greater power, cheerfulness, pride and functionality to address a few aspect.

FOR STRESS

4-7-eight Breathing (for relaxation)

Sit with no trouble.

Inhale thru your nostril for four seconds.

Hold your breath for 7 seconds.

Exhale for eight seconds.

Repeat.

This relaxes your involved device, slows coronary heart rate down and calms you.

Rhythmic Movement

Try a rocking chair, playground swing or a hammock to gently swing.

You can also roll a ball backward and forward rhythmically, or leap a ball in your lap, or just shift your weight from side to side fame or sitting.

You can start slowly and boom the depth as you want.

Reduces pressure, lowers blood strain and respiratory and allows you sleep higher.

Chapter 12: The Three Levels Of The Autonomic Nervous System

Overview of the Autonomic Nervous System

The autonomic worried system (ANS) is a branch of the worried device that controls the involuntary physical talents that we do no longer consciously manipulate, in conjunction with coronary coronary heart rate, breathing, digestion, and blood pressure. The ANS plays a critical characteristic in regulating physiological responses to pressure and social interaction, and it is accountable for maintaining homeostasis within the body.

The ANS is split into branches: the sympathetic worried tool (SNS) and the parasympathetic frightened system (PNS). The SNS is liable for the "combat or flight" response, that is activated in reaction to perceived chance or risk. The SNS triggers the release of adrenaline and special pressure hormones, causing the coronary heart price to increase, breathing to become faster, and blood vessels to dilate, bearing in mind extended blood flow to the muscle tissues. These physiological responses put together the body to reply to the perceived hazard, either with the aid of preventing or fleeing.

The PNS, alternatively, is accountable for the "relaxation and digest" reaction, this is activated at the same time as the frame is in a kingdom of relaxation. The PNS slows down the heart rate, breathing, and digestion, allowing the body to maintain energy and recover from strain.

The Three Levels of the Autonomic Nervous System

The Polyvagal Theory proposes that the ANS has 3 superb ranges, each with its very private particular set of physiological responses.

These tiers are:

1. The dorsal vagal complicated: This is the maximum primitive diploma of the ANS, and it's far liable for the "freeze" response. This reaction is activated on the equal time because the body perceives excessive hazard,

and it's far characterized with the aid of a lower in coronary coronary coronary heart price, respiration, and blood strain. This reaction is also related to dissociation and disconnection from the surroundings.

2. The sympathetic worried system: This is the second degree of the ANS, and it's far accountable for the "fight or flight" response. This reaction is activated at the equal time as the body perceives a moderate diploma of danger, and it's far characterised via an boom in coronary coronary heart price, breathing, and blood pressure. The sympathetic involved device prepares the body to reply to the perceived chance, each with the aid of using combating or fleeing.

3. The ventral vagal complicated: This is the maximum superior and sophisticated level of the ANS, and it's far liable for the "social engagement" reaction. This reaction is activated at the same time as the body perceives protection and reference to others, and it's far characterised by way of a lower in

coronary heart charge, respiration, and blood pressure. The ventral vagal complex promotes social conduct and conversation, and it allows for effective emotional law.

Understanding the three tiers of the ANS is essential for knowledge how our physiological responses are regulated in response to strain and social interaction. The subsequent chapters will discover each stage of the ANS in extra detail, similarly to strategies for regulating the ANS and using the Polyvagal Theory in every day life.

Description of the three levels of the Autonomic Nervous System

The Polyvagal Theory proposes that the autonomic worried device (ANS) has 3 outstanding degrees that adjust our physiological responses to strain and social interplay. These degrees are the dorsal vagal complex, the sympathetic nervous device, and the ventral vagal complicated. Each degree has its private unique set of physiological responses and behavioral results.

1. The Dorsal Vagal Complex

The dorsal vagal complex is the maximum primitive degree of the ANS, and it is liable for the "freeze" response. This response is activated at the same time as the frame perceives excessive danger or danger, and it's miles characterised thru a lower in coronary heart price, respiratory, and blood strain. The dorsal vagal complex shuts down non-vital bodily functions, which includes digestion, if you want to preserve strength for survival. This response is likewise related to dissociation and disconnection from the surroundings, which could reason emotions of numbness and detachment.

The dorsal vagal complicated is also associated with the parasympathetic tense system, mainly the dorsal vagus nerve. This nerve is chargeable for regulating the internal organs, at the side of the coronary coronary heart, lungs, and digestive device. Activation of the dorsal vagus nerve can result in signs and symptoms and signs together with fainting, gastrointestinal misery, and issue respiration.

2. The Sympathetic Nervous System

The sympathetic apprehensive device is the second stage of the ANS, and it's miles answerable for the "fight or flight" reaction. This response is activated even as the body perceives a mild degree of hazard or chance, and it is characterized via an boom in coronary heart rate, breathing, and blood strain. The sympathetic annoying machine prepares the body to reply to the perceived risk, every thru preventing or fleeing. This reaction is associated with the release of adrenaline and one-of-a-kind stress hormones, that can cause signs and signs and symptoms such as sweating, shaking, and progressed muscle tension.

The sympathetic apprehensive tool is also associated with the "typically will be inclined and befriend" response, that could be a social reaction to strain that consists of seeking useful resource from others. This response is greater common in girls than men and is idea to sell social bonding and connection.

three. The Ventral Vagal Complex

The ventral vagal complicated is the most evolved and complex diploma of the ANS, and it's far accountable for the "social engagement" response. This reaction is activated even as the body perceives protection and reference to others, and it's miles characterized with the aid of a lower in heart fee, respiratory, and blood pressure. The ventral vagal complex promotes social behavior and conversation, and it permits for effective emotional regulation.

Activation of the ventral vagal complicated is related to the discharge of oxytocin, a hormone that promotes social bonding and connection. This reaction is likewise related to the parasympathetic worrying device, in particular the ventral vagus nerve, which regulates the coronary coronary heart, lungs, and digestive gadget.

Understanding the 3 levels of the ANS is critical for know-how how our physiological responses are regulated in response to stress and social interplay. By information those responses, people can boom strategies for regulating their ANS and selling trendy properly-being. The next chapters will discover techniques for regulating the ANS and making use of the Polyvagal Theory in every day life.

Role of the Vagus Nerve

The vagus nerve performs a critical role inside the regulation of the autonomic worried gadget and is critical to the Polyvagal Theory. The vagus nerve is the longest cranial nerve and is liable for regulating many bodily abilities, which includes digestion, coronary heart price, and respiration.

The vagus nerve is break up into branches, the dorsal vagus nerve and the ventral vagus nerve. The dorsal vagus nerve is associated with the dorsal vagal complicated and is liable for the "freeze" response. Activation of the dorsal vagus nerve can cause signs and symptoms which embody fainting, gastrointestinal misery, and trouble respiratory.

The ventral vagus nerve is related to the ventral vagal complex and is responsible for the "social engagement" reaction. Activation of the ventral vagus nerve promotes social behavior and verbal exchange, and it permits for powerful emotional law. The ventral vagus nerve is also related to the release of oxytocin, a hormone that promotes social bonding and connection.

The function of the vagus nerve within the law of the autonomic traumatic gadget is complex and multifaceted. The vagus nerve has each efferent and afferent pathways, which means it may every send signs from the mind to the body and accumulate indicators from the body yet again to the mind. This bidirectional communication allows for the regulation of many physiological responses and behaviors, together with coronary coronary coronary heart fee variability, respiration, and emotional regulation.

One approach for regulating the vagus nerve is thru deep respiration wearing occasions. Slow, rhythmic respiratory can stimulate the vagus nerve and sell the activation of the ventral vagal complex. Other strategies for regulating the vagus nerve encompass meditation, yoga, and physical contact.

Understanding the position of the vagus nerve in the law of the autonomic worried gadget is critical for the usage of the Polyvagal Theory in every day lifestyles. By mission techniques that sell vagal law, human beings can enhance their emotional law, reduce pressure and tension, and promote everyday nicely-being.

Chapter 13: The Polyvagal Theory And Stress

Response to strain thru the Autonomic Nervous System

The Polyvagal Theory offers a framework for knowledge the location of the autonomic anxious device in our reaction to strain. The autonomic worried system is accountable for regulating many bodily talents, at the side of coronary coronary heart fee, breathing, and digestion. When we enjoy pressure, the autonomic nerve-racking device responds via manner of using activating the sympathetic concerned tool, which triggers the "combat or flight" response.

The combat or flight response is an evolutionary version that prepares our our bodies to reply to perceived threats. When the sympathetic concerned machine is activated, our heart price will boom, our respiratory will become speedy and shallow, and blood is redirected from nonessential organs to the muscle businesses, getting organized us for action.

However, at the same time as strain becomes chronic or overwhelming, the autonomic fearful tool can come to be dysregulated, essential to lots of horrific bodily and emotional signs and symptoms. Chronic activation of the sympathetic frightened machine can bring about improved coronary coronary heart rate variability, digestive problems, sleep disturbances, and an prolonged threat of growing chronic ailments.

The Polyvagal Theory offers a deeper information of the autonomic hectic tool's response to pressure, suggesting that the vagus nerve plays a critical function in regulating our pressure response. The ventral vagal complicated is answerable for the "social engagement" response, this is important for effective emotional regulation and pressure manipulate. When we feel constant and related to others, the ventral vagal complex is activated, principal to a sense of calm and well-being.

In evaluation, whilst we experience threatened or risky, the dorsal vagal complicated is activated, major to the "freeze" reaction. Activation of the dorsal vagal complicated can purpose symptoms and signs along side dissociation, numbness, and a enjoy of being disconnected from the frame and the surroundings.

Understanding the Polyvagal Theory can assist us extend extra powerful techniques for managing pressure and promoting emotional regulation. By sporting out strategies that sell vagal law, along with deep respiration bodily sports, meditation, and physical touch, we are capable of set off the ventral vagal complex and promote a sense of safety and connection, even inside the face of pressure and adversity.

Impact of strain at the frame

Stress is an inevitable part of lifestyles, and at the equal time as brief-time period strain can be beneficial, persistent or overwhelming stress may want to have massive terrible effects at the frame. When we revel in strain, our our our bodies reply thru freeing hormones which consist of cortisol and adrenaline, which put together us for movement. However, prolonged or continual publicity to strain hormones could have various negative bodily and emotional effects.

One of the number one impacts of stress on the body is advanced contamination. Chronic strain can reason an overactive immune reaction, which could make a contribution to the improvement of persistent inflammation. Chronic infection has been related to quite a number of health troubles, which encompass cardiovascular sickness, diabetes, and melancholy.

Stress also can have a massive effect on the cardiovascular tool. Prolonged exposure to strain hormones can bring about stepped forward blood stress, that might contribute to the improvement of excessive blood strain and precise cardiovascular troubles. Stress can also contribute to the improvement of atherosclerosis, a situation in which the arteries become narrowed and hardened, growing the risk of coronary coronary coronary heart assault and stroke.

Chronic strain can also effect the digestive device, fundamental to signs and symptoms and signs and symptoms and signs and symptoms which encompass diarrhea, constipation, and stomach pain. Stress can also contribute to the development of gastrointestinal problems which consist of irritable bowel syndrome (IBS) and inflammatory bowel illness (IBD).

In addition to those bodily outcomes, strain also can have a tremendous effect on intellectual fitness. Chronic pressure has been associated with the improvement of tension and melancholy, and it could moreover impact cognitive function, memory, and recognition.

Understanding the impact of pressure at the frame is crucial for developing effective strategies for coping with strain and promoting not unusual fitness and well-being. By undertaking strategies that sell vagal regulation and emotional regulation, such as deep respiration sports activities sports, mindfulness practices, and physical touch, we are able to lessen the terrible impact of pressure at the body and sell maximum suitable bodily and emotional fitness.

Understanding the Polyvagal Theory as a reaction to stress

The Polyvagal Theory gives a very unique and powerful framework for knowledge how we respond to strain. According to the concept, our autonomic involved tool has superior to reply to strain in 3 remarkable strategies, counting on the quantity of risk we apprehend.

When we apprehend a low diploma of hazard, our autonomic demanding system activates the ventral vagal complex, this is responsible for the "social engagement" reaction. This reaction is characterised by means of the use of emotions of protection, calm, and connection, and it allows us to engage in powerful emotional regulation and pressure manage.

When we apprehend a moderate level of risk, our autonomic fearful system activates the sympathetic concerned device, which triggers the "fight or flight" reaction. This response is characterized via elevated coronary heart charge, rapid breathing, and a redirection of blood go with the flow from nonessential organs to the muscle tissues, making organized us for movement.

When we recognize a immoderate degree of danger, our autonomic apprehensive tool turns on the dorsal vagal complicated, which triggers the "freeze" reaction. This reaction is characterised with the aid of emotions of dissociation, numbness, and a experience of being disconnected from the body and the environment.

Understanding those 3 responses to pressure can assist us expand extra powerful strategies for dealing with stress and promoting emotional law. By sporting out strategies that promote vagal regulation, at the facet of deep breathing carrying events, meditation, and physical touch, we are capable of prompt the ventral vagal complicated and sell a experience of protection and connection, even in the face of strain and adversity.

Additionally, information the Polyvagal Theory can help us apprehend at the same time as we're experiencing the fight or flight or freeze response and enlarge techniques for handling the ones responses. For instance, even as we are experiencing the fight or flight reaction, we are able to have interaction in bodily interest or rest techniques to assist regulate our respiratory and coronary coronary heart price. When we are experiencing the freeze reaction, we can interact in grounding techniques, on the facet of deep respiratory and physical touch, to help us reconnect with our our bodies and the surroundings.

Overall, the Polyvagal Theory affords a effective and complete framework for know-how how we reply to strain and growing powerful strategies for handling pressure and promoting emotional law. By information the role of the autonomic worried system in our reaction to pressure and attractive in strategies that sell vagal regulation, we're able to promote pinnacle-pleasant physical and emotional health and nicely-being.

Chapter 14: Trauma

How trauma affects the Autonomic Nervous System

Trauma may additionally moreover has a profound and lasting impact at the Autonomic Nervous System, especially at the capability to adjust and reply to pressure. When we revel in trauma, our autonomic concerned device can grow to be dysregulated, critical to chronic activation of the sympathetic involved tool and/or the dorsal vagal complicated.

Chronic activation of the sympathetic involved device can result in quite a number of bodily and emotional signs and symptoms and symptoms, which consist of prolonged coronary heart rate, fast breathing, anxiety, and hypervigilance. Additionally, chronic activation of the sympathetic worrying system can cause the development of persistent irritation and cardiovascular issues, similarly to digestive and immune gadget dysregulation.

Chronic activation of the dorsal vagal complex, on the other hand, can bring about emotions of dissociation, numbness, and a sense of being disconnected from the frame and the surroundings. This can result in a variety of emotional signs and symptoms and symptoms, together with melancholy, anxiety, and a enjoy of being disconnected from others.

The impact of trauma at the Autonomic Nervous System also can impact the functionality to adjust emotions and reply effectively to pressure. When our Autonomic Nervous System is dysregulated, we can also conflict to interact in effective emotional law and pressure control techniques, that would make a contribution to the development of persistent stress and horrible health results.

Understanding the effect of trauma at the Autonomic Nervous System is essential for growing effective techniques for trauma recovery and promoting perfect health and well-being. By sporting out strategies that promote vagal law, in conjunction with deep breathing physical activities, mindfulness practices, and bodily touch, we will prompt the ventral vagal complicated and promote a feel of safety and connection, even in the face of trauma and adversity.

Additionally, trauma-informed remedy alternatives, which incorporates Eye Movement Desensitization and Reprocessing (EMDR) and somatic experiencing, can help humans re-modify their Autonomic Nervous System and extend powerful techniques for dealing with the impact of trauma at the body and thoughts.

Overall, the Polyvagal Theory gives a effective framework for records the impact of trauma on the Autonomic Nervous System and developing powerful strategies for trauma restoration and most beneficial health and nicely-being. By carrying out strategies that promote vagal regulation and looking for trauma-knowledgeable care, humans can boom effective techniques for handling the effect of trauma at the body and thoughts and promoting lasting restoration and resilience.

The characteristic of the Vagus Nerve in trauma response

The Vagus Nerve plays a important feature in the body's reaction to trauma, as it's miles liable for regulating the Autonomic Nervous System and selling a enjoy of safety and connection. The Vagus Nerve includes branches: the dorsal vagal complicated and the ventral vagal complex.

The dorsal vagal complex is answerable for the frame's maximum primitive response to danger, called the freeze reaction. When activated, the dorsal vagal complicated can purpose the body to shut down, predominant to feelings of dissociation and disconnection. This reaction may be especially commonplace in individuals who've expert trauma, because the body's response to overwhelming stress and chance can reason the activation of the dorsal vagal complicated.

In assessment, the ventral vagal complex is chargeable for selling feelings of protection and connection, and is activated on the same time as people sense steady and constant. When the ventral vagal complicated is activated, people experience a revel in of calm and connection, which may be particularly beneficial for human beings who've professional trauma.

However, when the Vagus Nerve is dysregulated, humans may additionally moreover moreover warfare to activate the ventral vagal complicated and can enjoy continual activation of the sympathetic annoying machine and/or the dorsal vagal complex. This can result in pretty some of physical and emotional signs and symptoms, along with tension, despair, hypervigilance, and dissociation.

By carrying out techniques that sell vagal law, which consist of deep respiration physical activities, mindfulness practices, and bodily contact, people can activate the ventral vagal complicated and sell a experience of protection and connection, even within the face of trauma and adversity. Additionally, trauma-informed restoration strategies, inclusive of Eye Movement Desensitization and Reprocessing (EMDR) and somatic experiencing, can help people re-alter their Autonomic Nervous System and increase effective strategies for managing the effect of trauma on the frame and thoughts.

Overall, information the feature of the Vagus Nerve in trauma response is essential for developing effective strategies for trauma recuperation and selling best health and well-being. By conducting techniques that promote vagal regulation and looking for trauma-informed care, human beings can boom powerful strategies for managing the impact of trauma on the body and mind and selling lasting recuperation and resilience.

The importance of regulation in trauma healing

Trauma could have a profound impact at the Autonomic Nervous System, major to dysregulation of the frame's strain reaction and a number bodily and emotional signs. One of the critical element components of powerful trauma recuperation is law, or the ability to control and regulate the frame's response to pressure and trauma.

Effective law entails undertaking practices that promote vagal law, including deep respiration sports activities, mindfulness practices, and physical contact. By activating the ventral vagal complicated, human beings can promote a experience of protection and connection, even within the face of trauma and adversity.

Additionally, effective law consists of growing techniques for managing symptoms of dysregulation, consisting of hysteria, despair, and hypervigilance. This also can comprise growing coping techniques, which includes grounding strategies or self-soothing bodily sports, which could assist humans manipulate the effect of trauma at the frame and thoughts.

Trauma-knowledgeable recovery strategies, consisting of Eye Movement Desensitization and Reprocessing (EMDR) and somatic experiencing, also may be effective device for selling regulation and restoration. These treatment options interest on helping human beings re-alter their Autonomic Nervous System and increase powerful strategies for handling the effect of trauma on the body and mind.

Overall, the importance of regulation in trauma recuperation can't be overstated. By accomplishing practices that sell vagal regulation and seeking out trauma-informed care, people can develop effective strategies for handling the effect of trauma at the frame and mind and promoting lasting healing and resilience.

Techniques for Navigating Stress and Trauma with the Polyvagal Theory

Self-law strategies

The Polyvagal Theory gives masses of techniques that human beings can use to navigate stress and trauma. One of the maximum critical techniques is self-regulation, or the potential to manipulate and regulate the body's reaction to pressure and trauma.

Self-regulation techniques may additionally encompass deep respiratory sporting sports, mindfulness practices, and bodily touch, all of that could assist set off the ventral vagal complex and promote a enjoy of protection and connection. Other techniques may also additionally moreover consist of developing coping strategies, which incorporates grounding strategies or self-soothing bodily games, that may assist people control the effect of trauma on the frame and thoughts.

Trauma-knowledgeable treatment options, which includes Eye Movement Desensitization and Reprocessing (EMDR) and somatic experiencing, additionally can be effective device for promoting self-law and recuperation. These remedy plans recognition on helping human beings re-alter their Autonomic Nervous System and develop powerful strategies for coping with the effect of trauma at the frame and mind.

Additionally, humans may also additionally advantage from undertaking self-care practices, which includes normal workout, wholesome consuming, and good enough sleep, all of that can help promote normal well-being and resilience. Seeking social assist from friends and own family people, or accomplishing assist corporations or remedy, also may be useful in navigating stress and trauma.

Overall, the strategies for navigating stress and trauma with the Polyvagal Theory involve developing effective techniques for self-regulation, self-care, and searching for assist while preferred. By sporting out the ones practices, individuals can promote lasting recovery and resilience within the face of stress and trauma.

Mindfulness practices

Mindfulness practices can be a effective tool for navigating pressure and trauma with the Polyvagal Theory. Mindfulness entails the exercise of paying attention to the prevailing second, with out judgment, and with an thoughts-set of curiosity and openness.

Mindfulness practices can assist humans regulate their Autonomic Nervous System by activating the ventral vagal complicated and promoting a experience of protection and connection. By specializing in the cutting-edge moment and attractive in non-judgmental interest of 1's mind, emotions, and bodily sensations, humans can become extra attuned to their our our bodies and emotions, and expand more self-popularity.

Some common mindfulness practices embody:

1. Meditation: This consists of sitting in a snug function and focusing at the breath or a particular point of awareness, which encompass a mantra or visualization.

2. Body experiment: This includes lying down and bringing awareness to certainly one of a kind components of the body, noticing sensations with out judgment.

3. Mindful motion: This includes undertaking movement practices which consist of yoga, tai chi, or strolling meditation, with a focus at the triumphing second and physical sensations.

4. Mindful eating: This includes bringing recognition to the act of consuming, noticing the flavors, textures, and sensations of the meals without judgment.

By wearing out mindfulness practices, human beings can expand more self-recognition, modify their Autonomic Nervous System, and boom powerful techniques for handling strain and trauma. Mindfulness also may be used together with specific self-law strategies, together with deep respiration physical activities or physical contact, to sell a more feel of protection and connection.

Yoga and movement practices

Yoga and movement practices may be effective techniques for navigating pressure and trauma with the Polyvagal Theory. These practices awareness on movement and physical sensations, and may help humans regulate their Autonomic Nervous System through activating the ventral vagal complex and promoting a revel in of safety and connection.

Chapter 15: Applying The Polyvagal Theory In Daily Life

The importance of self-cognizance

The Polyvagal Theory may be done in everyday lifestyles to promote self-interest, emotional law, and resilience inside the face of stress and trauma. By know-how the standards of the Polyvagal Theory, people can grow to be extra attuned to their very non-public physical sensations and emotional responses, and extend effective strategies for dealing with pressure and promoting well-being.

One vital element of utilizing the Polyvagal Theory in daily existence is developing more self-recognition. This includes becoming more attuned to at the least one's personal bodily sensations, emotional responses, and forms of conduct. By growing greater self-interest, human beings can emerge as greater adept at spotting the signs and signs and symptoms of stress and trauma, and might growth effective strategies for handling the ones responses.

Another critical issue of applying the Polyvagal Theory in each day existence is growing effective self-law strategies. This also can include accomplishing mindfulness practices, yoga and motion carrying sports, or deep respiration wearing activities to assist modify the Autonomic Nervous System and sell a more enjoy of safety and connection.

In addition, individuals can follow the mind of the Polyvagal Theory of their every day interactions with others. This also can contain schooling active listening, expressing empathy and facts, and engaging in supportive behaviors that promote a experience of protection and connection.

Ultimately, making use of the Polyvagal Theory in daily life requires a strength of mind to self-attention, emotional law, and resilience within the face of pressure and trauma. By growing effective strategies for handling pressure and promoting well-being, people can navigate the challenges of every day life with more ease and resilience.

Strategies for education Polyvagal Theory in every day existence

There are numerous strategies that people can use to practice the thoughts of the Polyvagal Theory of their every day lives. These strategies can help individuals modify their Autonomic Nervous System, promote emotional law, and domesticate a more feel of resilience within the face of stress and trauma.

1. Mindfulness practices: Mindfulness practices, including meditation or frame scanning, can assist people increase extra self-consciousness and adjust their Autonomic Nervous System. These practices include focusing one's hobby on the prevailing 2d, without judgment, and can help sell a revel in of calm and relaxation.

2. Yoga and motion practices: Yoga and exceptional movement practices, collectively with tai chi or qigong, can assist people regulate their Autonomic Nervous System and sell a more sense of properly-being. These

practices involve mild movement sporting activities and respiratory techniques, that could help sell relaxation and decrease pressure.

3. Deep respiration physical games: Deep breathing sports, which encompass diaphragmatic breathing, can help humans modify their Autonomic Nervous System and sell a more experience of rest. These bodily activities contain taking gradual, deep breaths, that may assist sell a experience of calm and reduce feelings of tension or strain.

4. Social assist: Cultivating supportive relationships with pals and family individuals can assist humans adjust their Autonomic Nervous System and sell emotional regulation. By spending time with others who offer a sense of protection and connection, human beings can experience more supported and higher able to control stress and trauma.

five. Self-care practices: Engaging in self-care practices, consisting of exercising, healthful consuming, and restful sleep, can assist promote typical well-being and resilience. These practices can assist humans adjust their Autonomic Nervous System and promote emotional regulation, and can be an important a part of managing strain and selling a revel in of stability in every day life.

Overall, there are many techniques that individuals can use to exercise the requirements of the Polyvagal Theory of their every day lives. By cultivating self-popularity, regulating their Autonomic Nervous System, and attractive in supportive relationships and self-care practices, human beings can promote large nicely-being and resilience inside the face of pressure and trauma.

Importance of searching for help at the same time as important

While education the principles of the Polyvagal Theory may be useful for managing strain and trauma, it's far vital to recognize that attempting to find expert guide may be important at instances. Trauma and stress can be complicated and tough, and it may be beneficial to are seeking the steerage of a educated expert who can provide more aid and resources.

Some symptoms and symptoms and signs and symptoms that it is able to be useful to are looking for expert assist embody:

1. Difficulty regulating emotions: If you're suffering to regulate your emotions, which includes feeling crushed or now not capable of deal with pressure, seeking out the aid of a highbrow fitness expert can be beneficial.

2. Persistent signs of trauma: If you've got got experienced a traumatic event and are experiencing persistent signs and symptoms which consist of flashbacks, nightmares, or avoidance behaviors, attempting to find beneficial aid from a highbrow fitness professional can be beneficial in dealing with these signs and symptoms.

3. Interpersonal troubles: If you're struggling to your relationships or having problem

connecting with others, seeking out aid from a therapist or counselor may be beneficial in enhancing your conversation capabilities and developing more healthy relationships.

4. Difficulty coping with each day lifestyles: If you are finding it hard to manipulate day by day life due to strain or trauma, on the lookout for beneficial resource from a intellectual fitness professional can be useful in growing coping abilties and techniques for handling each day life.

Overall, looking for assist from a professional professional can be an important a part of managing stress and trauma. By jogging with a therapist or counselor, humans can broaden abilities and strategies for regulating their Autonomic Nervous System, promoting emotional law, and cultivating a more experience of resilience and properly-being.

www.ingramcontent.com/pod-product-compliance
Lightning Source LLC
Chambersburg PA
CBHW051727020426
42333CB00014B/1193